W9-CPE-088

Maximize Your Medicare: 2020-2021 Edition

Maximize Your Medicare: 2020-2021 Edition

QUALIFY FOR BENEFITS, PROTECT YOUR HEALTH, AND MINIMIZE YOUR COSTS

Jae W. Oh, MBA, CFP

THORNDIKE PRESS
A part of Gale, a Cengage Company

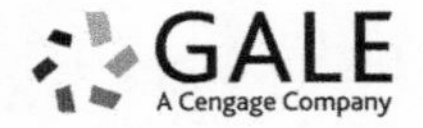

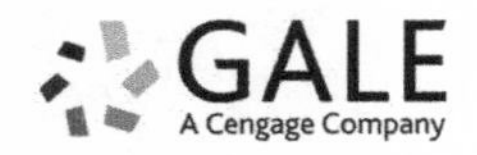

Copyright © 2020 by Jae W. Oh.
Thorndike Press, a part of Gale, a Cengage Company.

ALL RIGHTS RESERVED
Thorndike Press® Large Print Lifestyles.
The text of this Large Print edition is unabridged.
Other aspects of the book may vary from the original edition.
Set in 16 pt. Plantin.

LIBRARY OF CONGRESS CIP DATA ON FILE.
CATALOGUING IN PUBLICATION FOR THIS BOOK
IS AVAILABLE FROM THE LIBRARY OF CONGRESS

ISBN-13: 978-1-4328-7767-5 (hardcover alk. paper)

Published in 2020 by arrangement with Skyhorse Publishing, Inc.

Printed in Mexico
Print Number: 01 Print Year: 2020

TABLE OF CONTENTS

NOTE TO READERS: Premium levels, IRMAA premiums (part of Medicare Part B), and income brackets are subject to change per annual updates from the federal government. Always check for the most recent information, available here: http://www.maximizeyourmedicare.com.

INTRODUCTION

Medicare Is a Mystery: It Doesn't Have to Be

Medicare is enormous — there are about sixty million enrollees, according to the most recent Medicare Trustees Report.[1] That's about one in five Americans! As you might expect for such a vastly complex government program, its rules are confusing and frequently misunderstood.

For millions of Americans, misunderstanding the rules can mean unanticipated medical bills, overspending on prescriptions and health-care services, and other serious consequences. Health-care expenses are the number-one cause of household bankruptcy. And, as people age, out-of-pocket costs can overwhelm pensions, Social Security, and investments.

When understood and approached in the right way, however, Medicare is the single most valuable component of retirement planning in the United States, offering financial security, excellent access to health-care providers, and peace of mind. The regulations surrounding Medicare are heavily in your favor — but you have to understand the enrollment rules to reap all the benefits. In addition, fierce competition among insurance companies leads to very competitive pricing, which in turn means better benefits, lower costs, or both. You can use this information to set up Medicare in an optimal way — but doing that requires that you be fully informed.

That's the mission of *Maximize Your Medicare*: to make you fully informed. You will learn how Medicare actually works, how/when/why to enroll, and, most important, the crucial factors in choosing the best Medicare configuration for you and your family.

After countless presentations on the subject in addition to my consultation work, I can tell you that almost no one understands precisely how Medicare works. This is true regardless of education level, financial status, or profession. Everyone is liable to get his or her advice from people, including health-care professionals, whose information is inaccurate, incomplete, or outdated. This book will help you avoid these errors and get the most for your money.

This Happens

A highly educated, sixty-eight-year-old, very successful business owner is enrolled in employer-sponsored group health insurance. He is married, and the group plan covers him and his Medicare-eligible spouse. The premium of that insurance was $1,500 each, per month. Instead, they cancel their group health insurance and enroll in Medicare Part B (they had enrolled in Part A when they turned sixty-five), Medigap, and Part D.

Savings: $1,500, a month. Deductible: Lower by more than $5,000. Copays: None.

There are lessons to be learned here. First, this outcome was possible for the past three years. That is more than $50,000 of excess premium paid, for inferior coverage. That money cannot be recovered. One goal of *Maximize Your Medicare* is to inform you, so that you can avoid this combination of excess cost and inferior coverage. Second, it did not matter that this person was well-educated or wealthy — the misinformation delivered to him was still incorrect. The amounts can vary, but saving a few hundred dollars a year for a person who desperately requires every penny is worth the effort, and perhaps more so for a person that relies entirely on Social Security benefits for retirement income.

WHY IS MEDICARE SO IMPORTANT?

- Medicare can dramatically lower your health-care costs. There are a number of reasons this is true. First, premiums are much lower under Medicare, compared to individual health insurance, with superior coverage in most cases. The Medicare Advantage, Part D, and Medigap markets are very competitive. Insurance companies are competing very aggressively for your business, which works heavily in your favor. Second, your ability to enroll and make changes in the future is possible, if you understand that what you choose today can affect your ability to make changes in the future.
- Medicare has superior benefits. Under Medicare, access to health-care providers can improve. Medigap has no effective concept of network; the only limit is that the health-care provider must accept Medicare itself. Medicare Advantage has networks, but you can reasonably find a plan that includes most, if not all, of the providers that

you prefer. Medicare Advantage networks are now much more flexible than they were in the past. Some do not require a referral from a primary-care physician.

- Making mistakes can be costly. Errors in enrollment can result in penalties that may never expire. Not understanding the options under Medicare can result in you paying far too much for inferior coverage. These errors can limit your access to health-care providers, such as a specific specialist. The financial costs of how and what you choose can be many thousands of dollars a year. If a dollar saved is a dollar earned, then a dollar unnecessarily spent is a dollar wasted.

Why Is Medicare so Confusing?

- Medicare may look the same as other health insurance, but it works much differently. The choices you make today may affect the adjustments available to you in the future. This is a very important difference between Medicare and health insurance under the Affordable Care Act as it currently stands. For example, the words "deductible" or "network" may appear in both programs, but the practical implications of the words can be very different under Medicare.

- Enrollment rules are complicated. There is a huge difference between when you *can* enroll and when it is *best* to enroll. This is complex and becoming even more difficult for many reasons. The simple example is that Social Security Full Retirement Age has risen and is now sixty-six, but Medicare eligibility has stayed the same: most are eligible for Medicare at sixty-five, not sixty-six.

  Retiree benefits, small employer, large employer, COBRA, spousal coverage: any or all these terms combine to make your best selection very complicated, as each situation will have a different set of alternatives. Medicare, combined with health-insurance benefits for employees (and their families), has created a very wide range of coverage and cost combinations. People are frequently working beyond sixty-five, and this trend is not going to change anytime soon.
- Medicare components are oddly named. Unlike health insurance for those prior to becoming eligible for

Medicare, Original Medicare has specific components: Parts A, B, C, and D. Within Medicare Part C (Medicare Advantage), there are commonly thirty Medicare Advantage Plans available, some of which include prescription drug benefits, and some that do not. Within Part D (prescription drug plans), there are usually another thirty stand-alone Part D plans available in every geographic location. Medigap also uses a lettering system to describe plans: A through N. Sound confusing? It is.

- Advertisements and publications are incomplete. Advertisements from carriers are not intentionally misleading or inaccurate since every advertisement describing Medicare Advantage and Part D plans is highly regulated. *Medicare and You,* the annual document published by the Centers for Medicare & Medicaid Services (CMS), is a description of benefits under Medicare. However, the advertisements do not shed any light on what is important when making decisions and provide no guidance about how to choose among a wide variety of options. Regulations ban direct comparisons among Medicare Advantage Plans and Part D plans, so the advertisements and sales presentations are not wrong, but they do not provide the information required to make the best choices.

- There are changes every year. Numerous changes, both gradual and sudden, affect the Medicare eligible. Premiums and copays for Original Medicare (Part A and B), and the late-enrollment penalties, are recalculated every year. Medicare Advantage continues to expand, and retiree plans continue to weaken or be entirely discontinued.

  Why? Well, as we noted, Medicare is staggeringly large today, with sixty million current beneficiaries, and 10,000 becoming newly eligible for Medicare every single day. This is creating enormous financial strain on the federal government, and there is no end in sight without a complete overhaul of the health-care system. The result is that the government, employers, and insurance carriers have to make adjustments. They are all doing so, every year.
- A single detail can change everything. The icing on this already-complicated cake is that since everyone's set of

priorities and resources is entirely different, one single detail can be different, and that detail can make an enormous difference in your decision, when compared to your spouse, your lifelong friend, or your work colleague. It is not the goal of *Maximize Your Medicare* to determine what is important to you. It is the goal of this book to help you determine what may be best, given your specific set of priorities and resources.

How to Use This Book

Maximize Your Medicare is your guide through the Medicare maze. Every Medicare-eligible person needs to take these vital steps:

- Understand the enrollment guidelines. If you do not enroll according to the rules, there are late-enrollment penalties that never expire. In addition, you will not be able to simply "turn the switch on" whenever you want. You will have to wait, and while you're waiting, you might need health-care services or prescriptions. That can be very costly: you may be uninsured, or you may be wasting money.

For those eligible for Medicare prior to turning sixty-five (which we'll talk about later), there are untold ripple effects. For example, if you do not have a prescription drug plan that is deemed to be "creditable coverage," you get hit with the Part D Late Enrollment Penalty. But you may be able to enroll in Medigap (depending on where you live) or Medicare Advantage, which would save you a great deal of money compared to an individual health-insurance configuration. In other words, if you are eligible for Medicare before you turn sixty-five years old, there are ways you can save a lot of money or get far better benefits.

It is not only those planning on retirement or turning sixty-five years old who are affected. Current Medicare enrollees, who may have been relying on Medicare for years, must stay up to date too. People may prefer to "set and forget," but practical reality has made this approach unworkable.

- Understand what options are available. Simply understanding the enrollment rules is not sufficient. Why? Because your choices today can have consequences in the future. Some choices can be changed easily in the future (Medicare Advantage and Part D), and some may not, because the carriers may have the right to decline your application in the future (Medigap), which would make adjustments difficult, if not impossible.

This is not a suggestion that you be insurance poor; I would never give that advice. Medicare premiums and out-of-pocket costs are lower than almost any other health-insurance setup. But the plans change. What is best today may not be best next year, and the difference can be huge — hundreds or thousands of dollars a year.

- Get your best Medicare configuration. Your individual situation can vary widely due to your personal history. For example, if you are employed or retired, married or single, or receive retiree health benefits, what you need to know is almost certainly different than what your friend or neighbor needs to know.

While you can apply by yourself, you may want an expert/agent/advisor to help you confirm that you're approaching your individual issues in the best possible way. But not all experts, agents, and advisors are equally knowledgeable about the plans in your geographic location. This book will show you how to find the professional who's right for you.

The bottom line is that you need to keep up to date. I provide updates, breaking news, and commentary on special situations on the official website for the book: www.maximizeyourmedicare.com. There are many other ways to get information too:

- *Maximize Your Medicare* Facebook page
- *Maximize Your Medicare* newsletter
- *Maximize Your Medicare* Facebook community (you need to apply)
- *Maximize Your Medicare* podcast
- *Maximize Your Medicare* YouTube channel

These additional resources will help you especially because it is very likely that Medicare will change. For example, www.medicare.gov is the official Medicare website, with a Medicare Plan Finder. This is an important tool, and there are instructions on how to use the Medicare Plan

Finder in order to help identify a Part D and/or Medicare Advantage Plan.

The Medicare website has evolved greatly, and it is likely that the Plan Finder will also change. These resources will provide guidance when new processes or procedures become available.

Knowledge of how health insurance works is unlike almost any other type of financial knowledge. Normally, information that only you possess, and keep secret, is to your great advantage. That is not the case when it comes to knowledge about health insurance. The reasons are complicated, but one important factor is that the cost of health care is very high in the US and that there are uninsured, or underinsured, persons who leave unpaid bills with health-care providers. Losses suffered by health-care providers need to be recouped. How? Higher prices for the next patient — i.e., you.

So use these resources in addition to the book. Share them too, and help others — as I said, almost no one understands Medicare.

AVOID MISTAKE #1

Do not wrongly confuse health insurance with health care. They are linked of course, but they are not the same. Health insurance is a financial contract where you, as the insurance policyholder, receive benefits under certain conditions. For example, if your refrigerator breaks and is beyond repair and you have purchased an extended warranty, you receive a benefit — a new refrigerator. In the same way, health insurance is a contract that assists you, the policyholder, to reduce out-of-pocket costs if you require medical services: the reduction in health-care costs is your benefit.

When you purchase an extended warranty on a refrigerator, the cost of the extended warranty depends on the value of the refrigerator. It's the same for health insurance. The cost of health insurance depends on the value of the benefit you receive. Again, the ripple effect is important: the cost of health insurance depends on the underlying cost of health care. That means health insurance, as a contract, does not address the underlying cost of health care in the same way that the cost of the extended warranty does not fix or address the retail price of the refrigerator.

You can frequently read or hear in the media that "health-care costs are excessively high in the United States," and that the fix is to change the way that health insurance works. However, you can see, from the refrigerator example, the two terms are not the same; changing the way that health insurance works may not change the high costs of health care. What matters to consumers, you, is that you understand how health insurance can reduce your overall costs. Medicare? Simply a very specific type of health insurance.

Probability and statistics determine price of health insurance, not your physician. Your physician is administering health care.

Failing to understand that health insurance is different than health care is at the root of a long list of problems, miscommunication, and distortion. (Politicians wrongly conflate them all the time.) For example, health-care costs cannot be brought down by tinkering with health insurance. Why? Because, among other things, the costs of health insurance have no impact on how much it costs to become a physician, which needs to be offset through physicians' salaries, which in turn help determine health-care costs. Another example — a physician is an expert at the material covered in *Gray's Anatomy.* Insurance is priced using financial calculations and statistics. Being an expert in *Gray's Anatomy* does not, by itself, make him or her an expert in the Black-Scholes formula.[2]

Every day, people who do not understand health insurance ask questions of their physician. That would be similar to you asking your auto mechanic about which auto manufacturing stock to buy.[3]

VERY BRIEF HISTORY OF MEDICARE

Medicare was established in 1965 as an amendment to the Social Security Act. The federal government has two separate revenue accounts — they can be thought of as different funding "pots" — to fund the different parts of Medicare. There is the Hospital Insurance (HI) Trust Fund, used to fund Medicare Part A. It is paid for through federal payroll taxes. There is an annual Medicare Trustees Report which provides an update on the financial status of the HI Trust Fund. Then there is the Supplementary Medical Insurance (SMI) Trust Fund, which funds Medicare Parts B and D. The SMI Trust Fund receives its funds from premiums paid by beneficiaries (you), and from the general budget of the US government. In other words, it is funded by taxes.

Why does any of this matter to you? Groundbreaking reform to the Medicare system will remain difficult because the HI Trust Fund has already been paid over time.

That means current Medicare beneficiaries are the primary recipients of Part A benefits. If you widely expand the number of people enrolled in Medicare, there is no other way around this: much higher taxes will be required, or the existing HI Trust Fund will be diluted, resulting in weaker Part A benefits.

You can observe in the media and in think tanks that the United States has a more expensive health-care delivery system than other nations. There is endless name-calling and finger-pointing about this from every corner of our society. Changing health care from an à la carte system (called Fee for Service) to one where there is a singular price sounds ideal but introduces a problem. Creating an integrated health-care delivery system will be very difficult, because there have been very few proposals on how to deal with the fact that the HI Trust Fund and the SMI Trust Fund are separate tax revenue "pots." Combining the two Trust Funds (HI and SMI) would be very complicated, and it will require legislation. Dramatically changing and widening Medicare will invite political controversy to our already-divided nation. The reason? The existing HI Trust Fund has already been funded by payroll taxes, and the number of those benefiting from a public option, Medicare for all, or increased Medicare eligibility will likely dilute or divert the existing HI Trust Fund. The common sense conclusion is that existing Medicare beneficiaries' money will be siphoned off to a much larger pool of recipients, unless the shortfall is made up via higher taxes.

An example will make this easier to understand. Let's say you require a joint-replacement procedure. You'll need an X-ray to determine that this is necessary. There will be some local anesthesia, a surgeon, a location, the support people, and then the rehabilitation. Now, with Medicare, each of these stakeholders is being compensated under different Parts of Medicare (Part A or Part B), which raises two basic questions. If care costs $50,000, who gets what? And how much of the $50,000 comes from the HI Trust Fund, and how much from the SMI Fund? A complete solution to this has been, and will remain, elusive.

The simple fact, as this illustration points out, is a lot of information and noise surrounds Medicare. *Maximize Your Medicare* is not here to solve political or budgetary challenges facing the US. This book has one, and only one, constituent: you.

Ignoring Medicare Noise Is Difficult

The goal of *Maximize Your Medicare* is simple, which is to help guide you so that you can get the most from the Medicare program. Every person is different, and every situation is different, so it is logical that the definition of "the most" will also differ from person to person. The complication is that everyone faces a blizzard of highly fragmented information, sound bites, and tidbits from a very wide variety of sources. Some are credible, some are not; some are politically motivated; some leave out a vital piece of information. It is daunting.

Identifying the factors that are vital to you starts with the basics of enrollment and Medicare coverage. From that point, the real work begins: how to choose, why you would choose, and what factors should be considered in making the wisest choice for your situation.

Chapter 1
Enrollment

Truths and Myths

Truth: Medicare eligibility is usually extended to US citizens and legal residents who live in the US for at least five years in a row (including the last five), when they turn sixty-five years old.

Truth: Your effective date for Part A, Part B, and Part D is usually the first day of the month that you turn sixty-five years old (with some exceptions for those with a qualifying disability, end-stage renal disease, or amyotrophic lateral sclerosis (ALS).

Myth: You can delay enrollment in Medicare for a while and enroll later, and Medicare will be immediately effective. That is not the case if you do not have other health insurance. You would need to enroll during a specific time frame, and your coverage would be delayed.

Truth: If you delay Part B and/or Part D

enrollment, there are Late Enrollment Penalties that never expire.

Medicare Eligibility

There are many different dates to be mindful of, with confusing terms. The list is long, and the terms all look the same. On top of that, people and organizations often use the terms improperly and inaccurately. That makes a difficult situation worse. *Maximize Your Medicare* will use the precise terms consistently so that readers will not be confused. Let's start with the base case.

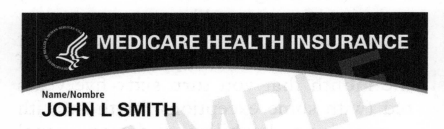

Initial Enrollment Period

The base case: The Initial Enrollment Period (IEP) begins three months prior to the first day of the month that you turn sixty-five years old. The IEP lasts for a total of seven months. The effective date is the first day of the month that you turn sixty-five years old. For example, let's use John L. Smith above. If John were born on March 22, 1951, then Medicare would be effective on March 1, 2016. John's IEP lasts for seven months, beginning on December 1, 2015, and ending on June 30, 2016.

First Exception

There is an exception to the date that Medicare coverage begins, which occurs for those born on the first day of any month. For example, John Smith could have been born on April 1, 1951. If that were the case, his coverage would begin on March 1, 2016, not April 1, 2016. The easy way to remember this situation? If you are a New Year's Day baby, your eligibility is December 1, not January 1.

Eligibility Prior to Sixty-Five Years Old

Some people are eligible for Medicare prior to turning sixty-five. Here are the situations when a person who is not yet sixty-five can be eligible for Medicare:

- Amyotrophic Lateral Sclerosis (ALS, or Lou Gehrig's disease). Patients are eligible for both Medicare Part A and Medicare Part B prior to turning sixty-five.

- End-stage renal disease (ESRD). ESRD patients requiring dialysis are eligible for Medicare, usually after receiving three months of dialysis treatments. If you have ESRD, please refer to the Glossary for a very important fact covering renal-disease patients. The challenge is to understand how to minimize out-of-pocket expenses under dialysis and is addressed in Chapter 8.
- Social Security Disability Insurance. If you are awarded Social Security Disability Insurance benefits, then you are automatically enrolled in Medicare Part A and Medicare Part B after receiving twenty-four consecutive months of Social Security disability insurance benefits.[1] One thing to note: military disability awarded by the Veterans Administration is not the same as Social Security disability.[2]

SIGNING UP FOR MEDICARE

Signing up for Medicare Part A and Part B is usually a simple matter. If you are already receiving Social Security benefits, then you will automatically get your Medicare card, and you will automatically be enrolled in Part A and Part B; in John Smith's case, coverage begins on March 1, 2016. You need not do anything else. Be sure that you actually receive your Medicare card. Anecdotal evidence is that it will arrive at the beginning of your IEP.

For others, you can go to the Social Security Administration, or enroll online at www.medicare.gov. For those with a special circumstance, a visit to the Social Security Administration office is recommended. If you are enrolling in Medicare because you are enrolling in Part B after the age of sixty-five, then a visit to the Social Security Administration office is recommended. In other words, online enrollment will work best for a base case, and only when enrolling as early as possible. It can take weeks from the time that you apply to the time that you receive your Medicare card.

Timing

For John Smith, let's look at the new card, and let's say his birthday is March 22, 1951. John Smith becomes eligible for Medicare on March 1, 2016. He can enroll in Medicare beginning on December 1, 2015, which is three months prior to March 1, 2016, his initial eligibility date. Remember that his effective date will not be until March 1, 2016.

John can choose to not enroll in Medicare Part B until three months after the month he turns sixty-five and face no penalty. He turns sixty-five in March. Add three months to that. If John has no other health insurance, then he can enroll in Medicare all the way up until June 30, 2016 without penalty. However, there is a separate Part D late-enrollment penalty, and if John waits until June 30, 2016, and has no prescription drug coverage, the Part D Late Enrollment Penalty will apply.

Very important note — if you wait until the month of your sixty-fifth birthday, or later, then your Medicare Part B effective date will be delayed by up to three months. For example:

If John signs up in March, then the effective date is April 1.
If John signs up in April, then the effective date is June 1.
If John signs up in May, then the effective date is August 1.
If John signs up in June, then the effective date is September 1.

Confused? The easiest solution is to enroll

during the first month that you can apply. These rules take precedence over all other Medicare enrollment rules, including any SEP, unless you were eligible for Medicare prior to the age of sixty-five.

Can I Delay Enrollment in Medicare?

I Work Full-Time; Can I Delay?

It is a very commonly asked, and often complicated, question: do I have to enroll in Part A if I am covered by my current/former employer? The answer is that it will depend on your employment status, the size of your current/former employer, and, in some cases, the employer's discretion. So, the answer is yes, you can delay, but that will depend on a number of factors.

The base case is that people usually enroll in Part A, because even if they are also covered by employer-sponsored coverage, Part A benefits can combine with existing coverage to lower out-of-pocket costs. However, it is complicated: this topic is addressed throughout Chapter 7.

As the workforce ages, and people continually work until later in life, this question will become more relevant, especially if Original Medicare cost-sharing details (deductibles, copays of Part A and Part B) weaken. The cost charged by employers to cover the Medicare-eligible employee and spouse is also rising; the terms and conditions of coverage may weaken. This combination has dramatically changed the decision-making process because it could be that voluntarily canceling employer-sponsored coverage is a superior option. Employers and employees routinely make very expensive errors when combining with Medicare.

That will depend on a long list of factors: the premium that the employee pays, whether or not there is a spouse or dependents covered under the employer-sponsored plan, the actual coverage terms, and conditions of the employer-sponsored plan.

Can I Delay Enrollment If I Retire?

If you and/or your spouse were covered by an employer-provided group plan and you retire and you are sixty-five years old, then you have an eight-month enrollment period in which you can enroll in Part B without penalty. This is useful information if your position has been eliminated, because then you may be eligible for COBRA. Mistakes are common here, because people try to play cute and delay enrollment until the last possible date.

COBRA Coverage: Should You Take It?

COBRA allows those who cease working for an employer to continue participation in group health-insurance plans.

COBRA can be used during the eight-month period when you can delay enrollment in Part B without penalty. It is not clear why someone *would* use COBRA, since COBRA premiums are much higher than Original Medicare, and, for those under sixty-five, the premiums are usually higher than plans under the ACA. There are exceptions: there can be reasons that you delay Medicare enrollment until the very end of the eight-month period. Here are two potential ones:[3]

- The prior employer-provided severance pays the COBRA premium.
- You have already paid the annual out-of-pocket maximum, or are approaching it, on your existing plan.

COBRA cannot be used as the reason to delay enrollment in Medicare beyond the eight-month period. Relying on COBRA beyond this eight-month period will result in the Part B Late Enrollment Penalty. To make matters more complicated, you will not be able to enroll until the following Open Enrollment Period, which runs from January 1 through March 31. Your actual coverage would not begin until July 1 of the following year, and the Late Enrollment Penalties would continue to accrue during the entire period, until July 1 of the following year.

For example, if you have relied on COBRA for nine months, and attempt to enroll in Medicare Part B on April 15, 2020, then you would need to wait until the Open Enrollment Period (January 1 through March 31, 2021), and your Part B coverage would begin on July 1, 2021.

LATE ENROLLMENT PENALTIES

There are actually three Late Enrollment Penalties:

Part A. You may be subject to a 10 percent Part A Late Enrollment Penalty, which lasts twice as long as the period in which you did not sign up but were eligible, if you enroll after the Medicare Initial Election Period ends. If you delayed, for example, for three years beyond the end of your IEP, then your penalty would be 10 percent per year for a duration of six years.[4]

Part B and Part D. There are additional, separate Late Enrollment Penalties for these, with separate calculations, and these penalties never expire. The calculation of the penalty is determined by the Social Security Administration.[5] These penalties can be waived if you qualify for Medicaid or if you qualify for Extra Help, the federal program to assist with prescription drug costs. The Part B Late Enrollment Penalty calculation is described in Chapter 3, "Medicare Part B." The Part D Late Enrollment Penalty calculation is described in Chapter 4, "Prescription Drug Coverage."

Some ask, "Why are there penalties?" The reason — insurance relies on a large population of people paying premiums, and not simply enrolling the moment they require health-care services. If every person in the population enrolled only when requiring coverage, then there would be no premiums from which to pay claims, and the entire system would collapse on itself.[6] Some people believe that providing funding is the role of the government, but that is a different topic, one that is left to public policy, not the rules of Medicare.

ACA Does Not Affect Medicare Enrollment

This fundamental question of whether ACA affects Medicare enrollment is raised by many, and the answer is not simple. First, the Affordable Care Act does not change Medicare enrollment or eligibility rules. The general cases described in this book will remain the same. There will be some changes to the decision-making process for those that are described in Chapter 7. If anything, those changes are subtle points about the timing and availability of choosing certain Medigap policies. The permanent "doc fix" that was enacted (called MACRA) does change the availability of choosing certain Medigap plans (Plan C and Plan F).

If you have enrolled in an ACA plan on the marketplace, whether that marketplace is offered on the federal or state-specific portal, you are not converted to Medicare automatically. In addition, you will not receive any notification from any party to inform you of your Medicare eligibility. There have been many errors in Medicare enrollment due to this misunderstanding. Lastly, you are responsible for canceling all health insurance when you enroll in Medicare.

Special Cases: Backdating Part A

Enrolling in Part A after the IEP can result in complications, even if you are covered by employer-sponsored group health insurance benefits. If your Part A application is filed more than six months after turning sixty-five, then your Part A coverage will be set retroactively to a date six months prior to the first of the month that you apply for Part A.

That introduces a special complication if you have Health Savings Accounts (HSAs), because you cannot deposit funds into an HSA while covered by Part A. This means that if you contributed to an HSA account after the date that coverage under Part A begins, you may need to contact your accountant to fully understand the tax ramifications.

In the future, this situation will become more common, as HSA-eligible health-insurance options are increasing in popularity, and people continue to work after reaching sixty-five. There are potentially unintended tax consequences for those that have contributed to HSAs.

Special Cases: Canceling Employer Coverage

Let's say that you are covered by your spouse's employer-sponsored plan and that your spouse works at a large employer. You delay Part B, which is allowed without penalty. However, upon your spouse's retirement, the IEP rules (see the delays mentioned earlier) will apply. Then it does become very complicated.

For example, Sherry S. turns sixty-five on March 15, 2019, and is covered by her husband's large-employer-sponsored health-insurance benefits. Her husband retires on May 2, 2019. Sherry's Part B will be delayed according to the IEP rules stated earlier. Her Part B coverage does not start on June 1, 2019; instead, it will begin on July 1, 2019. This gets very complicated when the cancellation of an employer-sponsored health-insurance plan occurs at the same time as the IEP, for either the employee or the spouse.[7]

MEDICAID

If you cannot afford to pay Part A and/or Part B premiums, then you should contact your state's Medicaid Administrator, a branch of the Department of Health & Human Services (the exact name will vary by state). Medicaid is a broad term, and there are three categories: Qualified Medicare Beneficiary Program (QMB), Specified Low-Income Medicare Beneficiary Program (SLMB), and Qualified Individual Program (QI). Each program has different income-level and financial-resource-level tests, based on the federal poverty level. Depending upon the program, assistance is available toward premiums, copays, and deductibles. Specific states can waive portions of the general guidelines, and each state has its own separate rules in determining whether or not you qualify.

There is a separate assistance program for prescription drug benefits assistance, called Extra Help. This was previously known as the Limited Income Subsidy (LIS), and that term is still frequently used. This is described in Chapter 4.

If you qualify for any of these programs, then you are allowed to change your Medicare Advantage or Medicare Part D plan once a quarter for the first three quarters of the year, because you qualify for a SEP as a recipient of financial assistance under these programs. The implication is that participation in these programs allows a person to ignore all annual enrollment periods.[8]

Conclusions: Thinking Ahead is Key

Enrollment rules are confusing, and not fully understanding them can result in penalties or delayed coverage. As a rule of thumb, the Medicare enrollment rules should be reviewed and understood at the earliest of the following dates:

- One year prior to the date that you would like to retire
- One year prior to turning sixty-five
- One year prior to your spouse turning sixty-five

Can the rules be understood in less than a year? Yes, certainly. However, there are moving components that you do not control. For example, your employer may have specific enrollment rules that require review. There is administrative red tape involved with both the Social Security Administration office and insurance carriers, which may require additional disclosures. So while the rules do favor the consumer, missing important dates should be avoided if at all possible. *Maximize Your Medicare* is not intended to increase hysteria; rather, it is to reduce the chance of you taking risks that you did not intend, and to reduce the chance that you are paying too much for the benefits you receive.

CHAPTER 2
MEDICARE PART A

NOTE TO READERS: Some of the figures mentioned in this chapter are subject to change per annual updates from the federal government. Always check for the most recent information, available here: www.maximizeyourmedicare.com

TRUTHS AND MYTHS

Myth: The Inpatient Hospitalization Deductible is an annual deductible. This is untrue. There is a separate deductible per benefit period.

Truth: Medicare Part A has no premium in most cases but has very expensive deductibles and copayments if you are hospitalized or require skilled nursing care.

Truth: Skilled nursing facility care and home health care are covered only if you have been admitted to a hospital, on an inpatient basis, for at least three days.

Truth: There is no annual maximum out-of-pocket limit if you have Medicare Part A alone.

Medicare Part A has the word "Hospital" next to it on the Medicare card. That is not a complete description. Medicare Part A and Medicare Part B can be considered to be the chassis, a starting point, like a foundation to a house. Misunderstanding this, and in particular, misunderstanding Part A, is one of the main sources of confusion regarding Medicare. This confusion over how Medicare Part A works leads to unanticipated bills, many of which could have been reasonably avoided.

Medicare Part A can be thought of as coverage for the cost of facilities. It is more than inpatient hospitalization.

A summary of the charges for Medicare Part A are provided in Table 1 at the end of this chapter (source: www.medicare.gov). Make sure that you know and understand the terms "deductible" and "copays" before proceeding. They can be found in the Glossary.

In most cases, Part A coverage can begin on the first day of the month you turn sixty-five. There are instances in which you can delay enrollment, and there are instances when you may be eligible for Part A prior to this day (see Chapter 1, under the section "Eligibility Prior to Sixty-Five Years Old").

Eligibility

The good news is that the price is zero, in most instances. You are eligible for Medicare Part A, premium-free, if you have paid income taxes for forty quarters (called Quarters of Coverage, QCs, by Social Security) and you have been a permanent, legal resident in the United States for five continuous years.[1]

If you are currently married for at least one year and your spouse is eligible for Social Security benefits when you turn sixty-five, then you will qualify for premium-free Medicare Part A. If you are divorced but were married for more than ten years, then you are covered if your former spouse is eligible for either Social Security or Social Security Disability Insurance benefits. If you are a widow(er), were married for at least nine months, and are currently single, then you qualify for Part A with no premium.

If You Don't Qualify

You do not qualify for premium-free Medicare Part A if you and your spouse have not paid Social Security taxes for the required amount of time, which is forty quarters. If this is the case, then you can pay for Medicare Part A yourself. It will be costly.

In 2020, Part A will cost $458/month for those that have worked zero to twenty-nine QCs. Part A will cost $252/month for those that have worked thirty to thirty-nine QCs. It is important that you contact your local Social Security Administration office in order to confirm your status.

You may be subject to a 10 percent Part A Late Enrollment Penalty, which lasts twice as long as the period in which you did not sign up, but were eligible, if you enroll after the Medicare Initial Election Period (IEP) ends.

You pay the penalty for twice as long as the period that you did not enroll. If you delayed for three years, for example, then your penalty would be 10 percent per year for a duration of six years.

Part A Benefits

This is a quick summary. A further explanation of subtle points follows.

Inpatient Hospital Stay

Deductible: $1,408 per benefit period.

First 60 Days: You pay $0. Medicare pays.

Days 61 to 100 Cost: You pay $352 a day.

Days 101 to 150 Cost: You pay $704 a day.

Days 150+ Cost: You pay 100 percent.

Skilled Nursing Facility Care* Stay

First 20 Days Cost: You pay $0.

Days 21 to 100: You pay the first $176 a day.

Days 100+: You pay 100 percent.

Inpatient Psychiatric Care

190 days lifetime benefit. Medicare pays 100 percent.

Hospice Care

$0 for hospice care.

You make a copayment of up to $5 per prescription for outpatient prescription drugs for pain and

*Skilled nursing care is a technical term and does not include solely custodial care.

symptom management.

You pay 5 percent of the Medicare-allowed charge for inpatient respite care (short-term care given by another caregiver, so the usual caregiver can rest).

Medicare doesn't cover room and board when you get hospice care in your home or another facility where you live (like a nursing home).

Blood

In most cases, the hospital gets blood from a blood bank at no charge, and you won't have to pay for it or replace it. If the hospital must buy blood for you, you must either pay the hospital costs for the first three pints of blood you get in a calendar year or have the blood donated.

Part A Inpatient Hospitalization Deductible

The negative with Medicare Part A is the large deductibles associated with Medicare Part A. The largest of these is the deductible that accompanies an inpatient hospital stay. For a hospital stay in 2020, the deductible is $1,408. For every benefit period (see "Key Term: Benefit Period," in this chapter), you are obligated to pay the first $1,408 of total hospital costs. The table at the end of this chapter shows the schedule of deductibles that you are obligated to pay if you are admitted to a hospital.[2]

The very high deductibles and copayments required under Medicare Part A are the primary reason that being covered solely by Original Medicare (Part A and Part B) should be avoided if possible (and it is avoidable in most instances). Any Medicare Advantage or Medigap plan, with prescription drug coverage, will be superior and potentially save you thousands of dollars if you are admitted even once to a hospital in any given year.

If you or someone you know suffers financial duress, then governmental assistance is available under the LIS (Limited Income Subsidy) or the Extra Help program, described in the previous chapter. Finally, there are Medicare Advantage Plans with no premium, which have all been approved by the CMS.

One other consideration is that the amounts of these deductibles and copays are determined by Medicare. They are subject to change annually. They are the source of annual debate and speculation. You don't need a crystal ball in order to predict which direction these amounts are going or how they will change over time:

they will be going up. It is a very large concern that the Medicare system is suffering extreme fiscal distress. One way to fix it? Raise taxes (Higher Income Related Monthly Adjustment Amounts can rightfully be considered a tax increase). Another way? Raise the cost-sharing responsibilities (deductibles and copays).

Outpatient Hospital Procedures

You may visit a hospital and be released on the same day. You may stay for one night and be considered to be treated on an outpatient basis. Even if the health-care services are exactly the same as if you were admitted on an inpatient basis, outpatient hospital procedures and all services administered during that time are not covered by Part A. If you are admitted on an outpatient basis, then the services received are covered by Medicare Part B.

The reason this is important is that the Medigap and Medicare Advantage handle inpatient hospitalization and outpatient procedures very, very differently.

Part A Copays

If you need to stay at a hospital for longer than sixty days, then the daily amount that you would pay with Medicare Part A would be $352 per day up to day one hundred. The copay amount would be $704 a day, between days 101 to 150. Beyond that, you are responsible for 100 percent of the daily cost.

KEY TERM: BENEFIT PERIOD

The Part A deductible is not an annual deductible. The key term to understand under Medicare Part A is "benefit period." This should be understood as a medical episode. For example, if you have a right knee joint replacement in January, you may be admitted to a hospital. Then, you will require rehabilitation, which may be done at home, or at a facility. Six months later, within the same year, imagine that your left knee requires joint-replacement surgery. This is an entirely new medical episode, a new benefit period, and you will be responsible for another Part A deductible.[3] You will owe another $1,408, and this may repeat for an unlimited number of times in one calendar year.

Now, it may be unlikely that you will have multiple benefit periods in a calendar year. Multiple hospital admissions within one calendar year is pretty bad fortune for a person, to say the least. However, it illustrates the fact that the deductible is not over the length of time (a year), you might normally presume. If you or someone you know has been admitted to a hospital and you have read an itemized hospital bill, you most likely noticed the cost of a single hospital stay will exceed the deductible. You will be required to pay the entire deductible amount per inpatient hospital admission.

Skilled Nursing Facility Care (SNF)

One very important point must be made clear: Medicare is not intended to be long-term care. It is not intended for use at a skilled nursing facility for extended periods. There are financial policies and contracts that exist to address this, and they are described in Chapter 9.

Since many skilled nursing home facilities cost more than $200/day,[4] you will most likely be required to pay the entire $176 per day for days twenty-one to one hundred. This type of care does not include custodial care, which is the care required for completing tasks such as grocery shopping and cooking.

A major change was introduced during November 2012. In the past, you were required to be making progress toward recovery in order to be eligible for Medicare benefits for skilled nursing care. However, since then, you do not have to meet an "improvement standard" to receive skilled nursing care benefits under Medicare Part A. For those afflicted by a stroke, or stricken with Alzheimer's disease, this is a very welcome change, since the condition may not improve, and yet, a patient may be eligible for Medicare Part A benefits.[5]

Observation Status

When you are admitted to the hospital, you can be admitted under inpatient or observation status. In order to receive Medicare Part A benefits for skilled nursing facility care, both of two criteria must be met:

You must have inpatient status.
The stay must last for at least three days (crossing three midnights).

However, if you are placed under observation status, then Original Medicare does not cover the first twenty days in a skilled nursing facility. In that case, the cost of skilled nursing facility care is not covered by Medicare Part A. The cost is covered by Medicare Part B, which is very likely to result in much higher costs to you, depending on your Medicare configuration. Medicare Advantage, Medigap, or retiree health benefit plans may be effective in reducing out-of-pocket expenses.

Why the confusion over hospital status? Hospital systems are under pressure to reduce the number of readmitted patients. Why? The CMS penalizes hospital systems based on the frequency of hospital admittances. Therefore, hospitals are motivated to admit patients under observation status, not inpatient status. Studies of hospital practices, however, seem to suggest that this practice does not systematically occur.

On August 6, 2015, H.R. 876, the NOTICE Act, was passed into law. The law requires hospitals to provide written notice to patients that receive hospital services under observation status for longer than twenty-four hours.[6]

The Two-Midnight Rule

The Bipartisan Budget Act (H.R. 1314) formalized the Two-Midnight Rule. If you stay at a hospital and receive services (not generally including the emergency room) over two midnights, then you are presumed to have been admitted under inpatient status, not observation status.

This rule took effect for hospital admissions as of October 1, 2013. The implication of this is that if you believe that you have been billed in error in the past, then you may have the ability to appeal and have Medicare Part A provide coverage, retroactively. This does not mean that it will occur automatically.

While the exact timing of what constitutes when the period begins (and from when two midnights is measured) is confusing to say the least, this will be taken as a positive development. It is important to note that certain Medicare Advantage Plans cover skilled nursing care, even if not accompanied by a three-day inpatient hospital stay. This will be addressed further in Chapter 5.

No Annual Out-of-Pocket Limit

The good news is that there is no limit on the lifetime benefits received under Medicare Part A. The bad news — there is no limit to the amount of out-of-pocket expenses that you can incur under Medicare Part A. Since there are no limits to the number of benefit periods in a calendar year, that means that there is no limit to the number of inpatient hospitalization deductibles, or copays, during a calendar year.

TABLE 1. Medicare Part A (2020)

Hospital Inpatient Stay	Copays Days 0-60: $0 Days 61-100: $352 a day Lifetime Reserve Days: $704 a day Lifetime Reserve Days are 50 days that can only be used once in a lifetime	Deductible $1,408 per benefit period
Skilled Nursing Facility Care Stay	Copays First 20 days Cost: You pay $0. Medicare pays. Days 21-100 Cost: You pay the first $176 a day. Medicare pays the rest. Days 101+: You pay 100%.	Note: Only after a three-day inpatient stay at a hospital. Skilled nursing care is a technical term and does not include solely custodial care.
Inpatient Psychiatric Care		190 days lifetime benefit; Medicare pays 100 percent.

Chapter 3
Medicare Part B

NOTE TO READERS: Some of the figures mentioned in this chapter are subject to change per annual updates from the federal government. Always check for the most recent information, available here: www.maximizeyourmedicare.com

Truths and Myths

Myth: There is an out-of-pocket maximum limit with Medicare Part B. You are responsible for the 20 percent coinsurance amount that Part B does not cover, without limit.

Truth: Part B premiums will increase in 2020 from $135.50 to $144.60, as a result of higher health-care costs.

Truth: The Part B deductible is an annual deductible. For 2020, it is $198; the amount is adjusted by the federal government on an annual basis.

PREMIUM

The Part B premium is indexed to income. For most, the monthly premium is $135.50. If you earn more than $87,000 as an individual, or greater than $174,000 filing jointly, you can be charged more for your Part B, according to the schedule in Table 2, which is included at the end of this chapter.[1] The income used to determine whether you owe the Income Related Monthly Adjustment Amount (IRMAA) will be based on the modified adjusted gross income from the most recently filed income tax return. If you are assessed an IRMAA, you will receive a notice from the Social Security Administration.

In many cases, the Part B premium is deducted directly from your Social Security check. This is not a requirement. That is, you can instead receive a bill for the premium. In an increasingly large number of cases, direct billing is the only possible way to pay. This is the case for those that are not receiving Social Security benefits. In addition, you may have saved money in a tax-advantaged savings account, otherwise known as an HSA.[2]

ANNUAL DEDUCTIBLE

In addition to the monthly premium, there is an annual deductible, known as the Part B deductible. For 2020, this amount is $198 per calendar year. You are obligated to pay the first $198 for medical services received. As per the Affordable Care Act (ACA), a fee cannot be charged to you for your annual preventive-care checkup. Once you have met the Part B deductible in a calendar year, you are responsible for the 20 percent coinsurance amount, as well as 100 percent of the Part B Excess,[3] if it is charged.

There are a few important points to keep in mind. First, all the health-care services you receive must be deemed reasonable and necessary by the medical provider, Medicare, and Medigap (but not necessarily Medicare Advantage).

Before receiving a diagnostic exam or therapy, simply ask the provider if that exam or therapy is medically necessary. A confident, competent medical professional should not be offended by this question. If a medical professional becomes defensive when asked this, then you need to ask yourself some serious questions.

Second, the Part B deductible is based on Medicare's allowed charges, a concept discussed later in this chapter. So, if a service received has an allowed charge of $100 and the doctor charges you $115, only $100 counts toward the deductible.

Third, the deductible is defined by Medicare on an annual basis. All details (premiums, copays, and coinsurance) under Medicare are changed by the government every year, meaning they can rise or drop annually.

Coinsurance

Once you have met the Part B deductible, then you typically pay 20 percent of the Medicare-approved amount for Part B services.

Part B Coverage

The Centers for Medicare & Medicaid Services (CMS) has a long list of approved services.[4] The precise definition that is commonly understood can be different from how the CMS defines a specific service. In addition, confusion arises because the list of approved services is subject to change or limitations.

Generally speaking, Part B covers:

Provider services: Medically necessary services you receive from a licensed health professional, such as a physician. This can be the subject of confusion, as noted in the following sections.

Durable medical equipment (DME): Equipment that serves a medical purpose, can withstand repeated use, and is appropriate for use in the home. Examples include walkers, wheelchairs, and oxygen tanks.

Home health services: Services covered if you are homebound and need skilled nursing or therapy care. It is important to note that this does not include custodial care, such as bathing or cleaning, unless this help is necessary in relation to your illness or injury.[5]

Ambulance services: Emergency transportation, typically to and from hospitals. For Medicare Advantage members, there are limits to the cost charged.

Preventive services: Screenings and counseling intended to prevent illness, detect conditions, and keep you healthy. In most cases, preventive care is covered by Medicare with no coinsurance.

Therapy services: Outpatient physical, speech, and occupational therapy services provided by a Medicare-certified therapist. As subset of "provider services," this can be the subject of confusion.

Mental health services.

X-rays and lab tests.

Chiropractic care when manipulation of the spine is medically necessary to fix a subluxation of the spine (when one or more of the bones of the spine move out of position).

Select prescription drugs, including immunosuppressant drugs, some anticancer drugs, some antiemetic drugs, some dialysis drugs, and drugs that are typically administered by a physician. For example, cancer treatments and infusion therapy for other diseases can be administered on an outpatient basis, in an office setting. They are covered by Part B.

Coverage Details

The following is a partial list of those services that people believe are covered by Part B. However, misunderstanding or administrative error can combine to create confusion and result in an invoice that beneficiaries and policyholders do not understand. While not exhaustive, this list will point out certain, but not all, services that are commonly misunderstood.

To make it more complicated, a Medicare Advantage Plan or a company-sponsored retiree health plan may override the exact terms and conditions stated on the official Medicare website. Under all Medicare

Advantage Plans, the terms and conditions of coverage, and your costs, are determined by the Medicare Advantage carrier, at its sole discretion.[6]

A "Welcome to Medicare" preventive visit is a comprehensive screening. EKG/ECG, flu and pneumococcal shots, and referrals for other care are included. It is important to note that if your physician administers other services not included in this visit, you are responsible for the customary Part B deductible and copays. This can be the source of confusion. In addition, this is different from the annual "wellness" visit, and the annual "wellness" visit cannot occur within twelve months of the Welcome to Medicare preventive screening.

Durable medical equipment (DME) is covered by Medicare Part B, subject to the customary Part B deductible and coinsurance. This can be a source of confusion because the DME retailer must be approved by the Medicare system. Further, Medicare Advantage Plans almost always have a network of DME providers to limit your out-of-pocket costs.

Office visits and consultations can be confusing. This is surprising but illustrates that Part B coverage can be more confusing than it appears. For example, consultations to certain specialists and health-care providers might not be covered by Part B. Anecdotally, the consultation to physical therapy can be rejected by the CMS, but the actual physical therapy sessions may be covered.[7] In addition, certain consultations with specialists (that is, neurosurgeons) may not be covered, even if the actual surgery is covered. You may ask your health-care provider whether the consultation is covered in advance.

Laboratory analysis is covered by Part B. When you are admitted for an outpatient hospital service, you may require additional laboratory services. This *should be* covered by Medicare Part B without charge.[8] However, practical reality can differ substantially, because a Medicare Advantage Plan may have a stated copay for these types of services.

Mammograms are covered without charge once a year. Mammograms that are conducted more frequently than this are subject to the customary Part B deductible and copay. A referral is not required for the annual mammogram.

Shingles vaccinations are not covered by Medicare Part B (or Part A). They are covered under the prescription drug benefits plan, either by Medicare Advantage or Medigap.

There are no longer any limits to the number of physical therapy visits during a calendar year. However, a Medicare Advantage Plan or retiree group plan may impose limits that override this detail. A Medigap plan would cover unlimited physical therapy visits as long as they are deemed appropriate and medically necessary.

Even if this is entirely clear, beneficiaries can still encounter problems. First, all services to be covered under Medicare Part B must be ruled necessary and appropriate by the CMS. If your physician has administered a service that does not fit this standard, Original Medicare will not pay, and you will be responsible. If your service is denied, you should receive an Advance Beneficiary Notice of Noncoverage (ABN), which informs you that the service is likely to be denied. You do have the right to appeal this decision, but the process has multiple levels. You may need to receive legal counsel, depending on the seriousness and cost of the denied service.[9]

Second, the CMS is keeping track of whether you have met the Part B deductible. This is very important for Medigap policy-holders. Why? A Medigap carrier, an insurance company, has the responsibility to pay for the 20 percent or a portion, depending on your Medigap plan. Prior to fulfilling your Part B deductible responsibility, a Medigap carrier is not responsible to pay any benefits on your behalf.

It is very difficult for people to identify and distinguish these issues. For example, there can be delays by the health-care provider in submitting claims to the CMS. The CMS may outsource the accounting responsibility, and that is subject to error. Those errors can originate either from the health-care provider or the third party responsible for accounting. So you should carefully review your Medicare Summary Notice (MSN), which details the services you receive and the way these services have been categorized.

SOURCES OF PART B CONFUSION

Part B Late Enrollment Penalty

Let's now consider the case that you decide not to enroll in Medicare Part B during the Medicare Initial Enrollment Period. Let's go back to the example of John Smith, who was born on March 22, 1951. Now, say it is August 15, 2016. For every twelve-month period, John Smith will pay a penalty for every year that he does not enroll in Medicare Part B. You might think that he could have simply signed up, and Medicare Part B would be effective September 1, 2016, right? Wrong.

When you do not enroll in Medicare Part B during the IEP and have no health-insurance coverage, then the next time that you will be allowed to enroll in Part B is during the Open Enrollment Period, which runs from the beginning of January through the end of March every year. The effective date of coverage under Medicare will not begin until July 1 of that year, which means that John Smith will not be covered until July 1, 2017.

If you are a penalty-paying beneficiary, your first effective date of coverage under Medicare can only be July 1. You will need to check with your Social Security office to confirm the first date that Medicare Part B will be effective. To make matters worse, you would be charged a rate that includes a penalty for not enrolling during your Medicare IEP. This Part B Late Enrollment Penalty period lasts forever.

If you are penalized for late enrollment for Medicare Part B, there is still an important step to take. During the Annual Election Period, which occurs between October

15 and December 7, you can (and should) select a stand-alone Prescription Drug Plan (Medicare Part D, described in Chapter 5).

If you do not do that, there is a separate Part D late enrollment penalty, which will continue to accumulate until you have creditable prescription drug benefits. If this is the situation (no Part B, only Part A), then the only way to avoid additional Part D late enrollment penalties is to enroll in a stand-alone prescription drug plan during the Annual Election Period.

Part B Accounting

The CMS, besides keeping track of whether you have satisfied the Part B deductible, also monitors your Medigap, Medicare Advantage, and Part D provider (insurance company), if applicable. It is vital to know that the CMS is outsourcing the accounting of this function, and that errors can, and do, occur.

You will receive a Medicare Summary Notice (MSN) throughout the year. There, you will find the CMS's accounting of your progress toward meeting the Part B deductible. In addition, you can create an account at www.mymedicare.gov, where you will be able to track Medicare claims and obtain information about your Medicare coverage.

For Medigap policyholders, the Part B deductible can be very troublesome, because if you have not met it, or if the CMS has not recorded the fact that you have met the deductible, then the Medigap carrier, an insurance company, will not know either. Before you have met the Part B deductible, the Medigap carrier will not pay benefits, except in the case of Plans C and F.

Part B Excess

Once you have met the Part B deductible, then you have the coinsurance arrangement with Medicare. Medicare will pay for 80 percent of approved, medically necessary services. You will be obligated to pay for the remaining 20 percent. If you require surgery, and the physician charges $30,000, then you will owe at least $6,000.

Could you owe more than $6,000, even when that is 20 percent of the total cost? Yes. It is very important to understand what this 80 percent and 20 percent mean. Medicare will pay 80 percent of the Medicare-allowed charge. What is the Medicare-allowed charge?

Key Term: Medicare-Approved Amount

Medicare has a long and extensive, almost exhaustive, list of services and treatments delivered by doctors or medical professionals. Each item has an amount to be paid to medical providers for that particular service. That is the Medicare-allowed amount. Presuming that the service is deemed reasonable and necessary, Medicare will pay 80 percent of the allowed amount, leaving you with 20 percent as an out-of-pocket expense.

Confusion often occurs when the doctor/medical provider charges more than the Medicare-allowed charge. A medical provider can bill up to 15 percent more than the Medicare-allowed charge. A number of scenarios can occur.

First, the doctor may accept the Medicare-allowed charge as full payment.[10] You will simply owe the 20 percent of the Medicare-allowed charge. However, the medical provider may not accept the Medicare-allowed charge as full payment. So, in addition to the 20 percent of the Medicare-allowed charge that the Medicare system does not pay (which you will have to pay), you will also have to pay the entire extra amount that the medical provider charges above and beyond the Medicare-allowed charge. The amount above the Medicare-allowed amount is called the Medicare Part B Excess. Confused? Let's try an example to illustrate this important concept so you can make a better-informed decision.

Part B Excess Example
This Happens

A doctor wants to charge $30,000 for an outpatient surgical procedure, and the Medicare-allowed charge is $27,000. In addition, let's assume that you have already satisfied the Part B deductible. In this case, the doctor can choose to take the $27,000 and accept that as full payment. However, the doctor can charge up to 15 percent more than the $27,000. In this example, let's say the surgeon chooses to charge $30,000.

Medicare will pay for 80 percent of $27,000, or $21,600, and you will have to pay 20 percent of $27,000, or $5,400. In addition, you will need to pay the entire amount that the doctor charges above the Medicare allowed-charge amount.

In this example, the Part B Excess is $3,000 ($30,000 less $27,000). Therefore, your out-of-pocket expenses would be $5,400 plus $3,000, or $8,400.

Total Bill = $30,000
Medicare-allowed charge = $27,000
Medicare pays = $27,000 × 80% =

$21,600, *not* $30,000 × 80%

You pay 20 % of Medicare-allowed charge:
$27,000 – $21,600 = $5,400

You pay the entire Part B Excess = $30,000 – $27,000 = $3,000

Your Total Cost = $5,400 + $3,000 = $8,400

There is an important exception to this. Certain states have laws that prohibit a medical provider from charging more than the Medicare-allowed amount: Connecticut, Massachusetts, Minnesota, New York, Ohio, Pennsylvania, Rhode Island, and Vermont. The law that prevents Medicare Part B Excess charges is called the Medicare Overage Measure Law (MOM).

If you think that you can simply move to one of these states in order to avoid this, anecdotal evidence strongly suggests that the Medicare-allowed charges in these locations are higher, and therefore, premiums are also higher for Medigap plans.

Specifically, Plan G will cost more than other Medigap plans, but if you encounter the Part B Excess, then the "math of money" can easily be that the benefits may exceed the difference in premium. In addition, health-care providers may not charge a Part B Excess today, but can do so in the future. Given the national health-care reform debate, and potential lower payment rates to health-care providers, charging the Part B Excess may be a logical, rational response by physicians and other health-care providers.

It is important to note that under almost every group plan, employer-provided plan, and Medicare Advantage (MA) plan (including MAPD), the Part B Excess is not covered. On the other hand, most Medicare Advantage Plans disallow "balance billing," which is charging the patient an amount above the amount paid by the Medicare Advantage provider to the healthcare provider. While the probability may be small, the potential financial effect can be dramatic. You need to carefully consider this point when deciding on the proper coverage under Medicare.

The benefit of having this paid, without worry, may be worth the extra cost. This is particularly true for those that have known medical issues when entering the Medicare Initial Enrollment Period. Under the existing Medicare system, beginning in January 2020, only Medigap Plan G and the new high-deductible Plan G will cover the Part B Excess. Those who are already enrolled in Medigap Plan F and high-deductible Plan

F are also covered. In addition, one type of Medicare Advantage, called PFFS, can result in no Part B Excess, because the medical provider has agreed, in advance, to accept the Medicare-approved amount as full payment.

Canceling Medicare Part B

Canceling Medicare Part B is a serious matter, but you can do it. There can be a justifiable reason to do so. For example, you may return to full-time work for an employer whose benefits plan does not require enrollment in Medicare Part B.

To cancel, you will need to go to your local Social Security Administration office and go through an interview. That will allow you to fill in the form CMS-1763. The SSA will not mail you one, and it is not available online. The reason is that if you attempt to reenroll, you may be required to pay a penalty. Then again, if you are canceling Medicare Part B to enter another health insurance plan from an employer, you can reenter Medicare Part B without penalty. The SSA wants to make sure that you understand the consequences. This is complicated and needs to be handled carefully.

NO ANNUAL OUT-OF-POCKET LIMIT

The good news is that there is no limit on the lifetime amount of benefits that you can receive under Medicare Part A or Part B. The bad news — there is no annual limit to the amount of out-of-pocket expenses that you can incur under Medicare Part A or Medicare Part B.

This has very powerful implications for financial planning and retirement planning. The notion that "I have my Medicare card, I'm all set" is incorrect because your financial liability, if you face a medical situation that persists, is unlimited. Thinking that Part A and Part B alone are sufficient cannot be correct, especially when you consider that some Medicare Advantage Plans (Chapter 5) can cost no additional premium and must include an annual out-of-pocket limit.

TABLE 2. Medicare Part B Premiums (2020).

Annual deductible is $198.00.

Individual	Joint	Monthly Premium
$87,000 or less	$174,000 or less	$144.60
$87,000 – $109,000	$174,000 – $218,000	$202.40
$109,000 – $136,000	$218,000 – $272,000	$289.20
$136,000 – $163,000	$272,000 – $326,000	$376.00
$163,000 – $500,000	$326,000 – $750,000	$462.70
Greater than $500,000	Greater than $750,000	$491.60

Source: CMS

Chapter 4
Prescription Drug Coverage

NOTE TO READERS: Some of the figures mentioned in this chapter are subject to change per annual updates from the federal government. Always check for the most recent information, available here: www.maximizeyourmedicare.com

Truths and Myths

Myth: You can have multiple creditable coverage prescription drug plans.

Truth: If you are eligible for Medicare, you must have "creditable coverage." If you are uncovered for any longer than sixty-three days, you will be subject to a Part D Late Enrollment Penalty. That penalty never expires.

Truth: You can obtain creditable coverage through stand-alone Part D plans, which are offered by insurance companies. Every Part D plan meets a set of set of minimum requirements, and many Part D plans exceed many of these requirements.

Truth: The calculation of your True Out-of-Pocket Costs (TrOOP) for prescriptions is not the same as the actual amount of money that you spend.

The Basics

Prescription drug costs account for more than one out of every five dollars spent by Medicare beneficiaries. There are a variety of ways that you can obtain prescription drug coverage when eligible for Medicare:

Stand-alone prescription drug plan. These are known as Part D plans. Nationwide, there are between twenty-two and thirty Part D plans available in every state.

Medicare Advantage Prescription Drug Plans. These are specific Medicare plans that include health and prescription coverage. There can be as many as sixty Medicare Advantage Plans available that include prescription drug benefits.

For veterans, TRICARE or VA drug coverage. For veterans, these plans qualify as creditable coverage. TRICARE or your VA provider should send you information to verify this.

Indian Health Service, Tribal Health Program, or Urban Indian Health Program provide prescription drug benefits which qualify.

Federal Employee Health Benefits (FEHB) program. Annuitants have prescription drug benefits that qualify as creditable coverage.

All statements that pertain to Part D in this book also apply to the prescription drug benefits that are embedded within Medicare Advantage Prescription Drug (MAPD) plans. The Centers for Medicare & Medicaid Services (CMS) will not allow you to have multiple prescription plans that fit the "creditable coverage" standard. In addition, if you do not have creditable coverage for more than sixty-three days after first becoming eligible for Medicare Part A, you may be subject to a Part D Late Enrollment Penalty, which never expires.

ELIGIBILITY

If you are eligible for Medicare coverage, you are also eligible for the Medicare drug benefit (Part D). You must be enrolled in Medicare Part A and/or Part B to enroll in Part D. This means that you could, in theory, be enrolled in the following:

- Medicare Part A, Part B, and Part D
- Medicare Part A and Part D only
- Medicare Part B and Part D only

Enrollment

For those that are newly eligible for Medicare Part A and Part B, the Medicare Initial Enrollment Period (IEP) applies. In our John Smith case from Chapter 1, he turned sixty-five on March 22, 2016. That means he could enroll in Part D plans as early as December 1, 2015, and as late as May 31, 2016, without incurring a penalty. The earliest that Part D coverage could begin was March 1, 2016.[1]

Part D Late Enrollment Penalty

After June 30, 2016, John Smith would begin to incur a penalty if he had not enrolled in Medicare Part D. The Medicare Part D penalty rate is 1 percent for every month that you do not enroll. The amount of the penalty is based on the national average of the price of a prescription drug plan, not on the 1 percent of the plan that you select. This penalty never expires; it lasts the remainder of your life.

Let's start with an example. Say you choose an inexpensive prescription drug plan. The penalty will not be based on your plan's premium but rather on the national average Part D premium. If the average drug plan costs $33.19, which is the 2019 average, then your penalty would be $0.3319 for every month that you did not enroll in the plan during your open enrollment. If you are required to pay a penalty because you delayed enrollment for ten months, you would be required to pay ten times $.3319 or a $3.319 monthly penalty, rounded to the nearest $0.10, which is $3.30 per month.

The maximum penalty would be calculated from June 1, 2006, the date that Medicare Part D originally began.

The total penalty will depend on the average Part D premium and is recalculated for every month that you do not have creditable prescription drug coverage.

Let's say that you are penalized for three months during 2018 and twelve months during 2019. In that case your penalty will be:

3 months × 1 percent × $35.02 (the 2018 average Part D premium) = $1.0506 *plus*

12 months × 1 percent × $33.19 (the 2019 average Part D premium) =

$3.9828 *equals*

$5.0334, rounded to the nearest $0.10 = $5 per month to be added to your Part D premium[2]

PRESCRIPTION DRUG PLAN TERMS

Premiums. Each stand-alone prescription plan has its own specific stated premium. However, premiums are also indexed to income, which means that if you earn more than $87,000 as an individual, or greater than $174,000 filing jointly, you can be charged more for your Part D or Medicare Advantage Prescription Drug Plan.

The additional amount is called the Income-Related Monthly Adjustment Amount (IRMAA). The IRMAA will automatically be deducted from your Social Security benefit. If you do not receive Social Security benefits, you are responsible for the plan's stated premium plus IRMAA. The IRMAA for Part D is found in Table 3 at the end of this chapter.[3]

Copays. Different copayments will exist for each drug, and they will not be the same across plans. That is why you may need the assistance of the Medicare website or an insurance agent. Paper copies of the formularies that itemize the medications covered by your MAPD plans are sent before the Annual Election Period to enrollees.

Formulary. Each plan will have a formulary, a list of medications covered by the plan, and the tier that specifies your financial responsibility. The specifications can be tricky, since the formularies can change within a calendar year. Every formulary will have at least two medications for each medical condition, as governed by the CMS.

Exceptions. If you have been prescribed a medication that is not part of the formulary, you can file a formulary exception. The Part D plan (or MAPD plan) carrier will have an exception request form, which must be completed by the prescriber's supporting statement.

Tiers. Every prescription drug is assigned a tier by the Part D or MAPD plan. These tiers are not the same across carriers or plans. The number of tiers may vary, and the medications within each tier will vary. In addition, a complication can arise because formularies can change during the year, in which case a specific medication can also move into a different tier.

Prior Authorization and Quantity Limits. Certain medications create financial complications due to their high cost. There are a number of ways that a Part D or MAPD plan may approach this: Prior Authorization, Step Therapy, or Quantity Limits. Your physician can provide a written explanation to grant Prior Authorization or to override Quantity Limits. Step Therapy means trying less expensive options before "stepping up" to drugs that cost more. In addition, if you have expensive medications you will need to work with insurance companies because the companies may expect you to participate in a therapy program to make sure that you are not taking an unnecessarily expensive medication for an extended period.

The Standard Part D Plan

Here are the terms of Medicare Part D (premiums *not* included): Every Part D plan must be at least as good as these guidelines. Your plans may exceed these standards; it will depend on the specific Part D or MAPD plan. For example, the specific Part D or Medicare Advantage Plan may have a lower deductible or coverage within the coverage gap (more on that later). That will vary from plan to plan, from year to year. It is important to know that each of these tiers is redefined, every year. Here are the terms of Medicare Part D (premiums *not* included):

$0 to $435: If the costs fall into this range in a calendar year, then the Medicare Part D is paid according to the plan that you purchase. Premiums, deductibles and copays vary by plan. Applicants should check on the website www.medicare.gov to find out which Medicare Part D plans cover the drugs that the applicant takes.

$435 to $4,020: You pay a copay or coinsurance of the total costs of prescriptions between $435 and $4,020. The Medicare Part D plan or your Medicare Advantage Drug Plan pays the remainder.

$4,020 to $6,350: In 2020, there is a 75 percent discount on covered brand-name prescription drugs and a 75 percent discount on the cost of generic drugs while in this gap. This has essentially closed coverage gap, also known as the "donut hole." What's important here is that certain stand-alone prescription plans provide for partial coverage inside the coverage gap (described later in this chapter). If you fall in this range and you know in advance that you will fall within the coverage gap, then it can be the case that you should choose a plan with a higher premium, which may result in lower overall costs throughout a calendar year. You should check this every year.

$6,350+ (catastrophic coverage stage): You pay the maximum of $3.30 or 5 percent of the total costs of generic and multisource preferred prescriptions above $6,350.[4] For preferred prescriptions, you will pay the maximum of 5 percent or $8.25. For generic medications, you will pay the greater of 5 percent or $3.40. The Medicare Part D provider pays the remainder. This is called catastrophic coverage.

THE COMPLICATED CALCULATIONS INVOLVED IN PART D

There are very subtle, important differences among the terminology used in Part D plans. The most important of these is that the out-of-pocket costs are not the same as total drug costs.

Out-of-Pocket Costs under Part D:

Does not include the premiums for the Part D plan.

Does include the discounts via the Extra

Help program.

Does include the discounts under the Medicare coverage gap.

Does include the discounts under most state Pharmaceutical Assistance Programs.

Are totaled to calculate the TrOOP, and those define the threshold of reaching the catastrophic coverage stage, as described in the prior section.

Total Drug Costs under Part D:

Does not include the premiums for the Part D plan.

Does include the copays and coinsurance prior to reaching the coverage gap.

Does include what the plan pays on your behalf. This means that there is a stated cost of a medication, let's say $100, and a copay of $20. So the plan is paying $80 on your behalf. Therefore, the entire $100 ($20 + $80) is counted under total drug costs. This is the source of misunderstanding when estimating whether you will reach the coverage gap.

Are totaled to calculate if you enter the coverage gap ("donut hole"). Does this matter? For those that never threaten the lower boundary of the coverage gap, this is not an issue. However, those with multiple medications, especially if there is a single expensive medication, may face the coverage gap and the catastrophic coverage stage.[5]

Why People Misunderstand the Coverage Gap

It is entirely understandable that people are confused by the Part D coverage gap. The primary reason is that the calculations as described in the prior list are not your actual amounts paid, but the sum of the retail cost of your medications and the discounts granted by pharmaceuticals.

For example, take levothyroxine sodium, the generic form of synthroid, which is used to treat hypothyroidism. Let's assume that you have a stand-alone prescription plan named "Acme Medicare PDP." Acme has negotiated a price of $30 for a ninety-day supply. Let's say that your copay, under the Acme Medicare PDP, for levothyroxine sodium is $15 for the ninety-day supply. In this case, $15 is what you will pay. However, the total drug cost calculation does not use the $15 copay for your calculation of total drug costs. Instead, $30 is the amount used to calculate total drug costs. The implication here is that you can reach the coverage gap sooner than you would otherwise believe.

Once reaching the coverage gap, pharmaceutical companies are required to offer a discount to you. Another example: Let's say the cost of a medication is $500, and the pharmaceutical company offers a 70 percent discount and the plan offers a 5 percent discount, resulting in an out-of-pocket cost of $125. However, the total cost of drugs used is $500, not $125. The implication here works in your favor, because it shortens the time that you would remain in the coverage gap.[6]

Important reminder: The monthly premium that you pay is not included in the total drug cost calculation.

How to Choose

Using Medicare Plan Finder

Once you have decided to enroll in a prescription drug plan, the question becomes what the best plan is for you. This will require some work on your part. You may request the assistance of an expert or a professional. You can do it yourself by going to www.medicare.gov. Here are the steps to take:

1. Click "Find Health & Drug Plans."
2. Choose "Continue without logging in." It is important to not login because doing so will allow all of your personal, private Medicare information to be viewed on your computer.
3. Choose "View plans. I know what type of plan I want."
4. Choose "Drug Plan (Part D)."
5. Enter your zip code and choose the correct county of residence.
6. Choose "no" under "Do you have a Medicare number?" While you can choose "yes," remember that this means you will be logging in, and your private, personal information, including claims history, will be viewable.
7. Enter your date of birth.
8. Answer "Do you get help with your costs from one of these programs?" It is an important step, so choose the correct option.
9. "Do you want to see your drug costs when you compare plans?" Choose "yes."
10. "How do you normally fill your prescriptions?" Choose "Both." Again, this is important because you are attempting to identify the lowest-cost drug coverage. It is not necessarily the

case that mail order is the least expensive.

11. Enter your prescription drugs. It is very important to enter the generic drug name, if you are using a generic form. Once completed, choose "Done."
12. Choose pharmacies from the list. When complete, choose "Done."
13. Find "Sort plans by," and choose "Lowest drug cost."
14. The results will be in order, with the least expensive plans listed first. Make sure you conduct this exercise multiple times, with different pharmacies, if many are available in your location.[7]

Important Hints on Using the Medicare Plan Finder

There are some important tips to keep in mind while selecting a Part D plan using the Medicare website. If you do not follow these instructions, the answers that you receive can be wrong.

First, use the generic name if the generic form of a medication is used.

Second, if you do not refill a prescription every month, make certain to adjust the dosage and frequency appropriately. This can be vital for expensive mediations. The sensitivity of the proper plan will usually depend on the expensive medication(s) that you are prescribed.

Third, if you have the ability to use many different pharmacies, then you can experiment with the website and use different combinations of pharmacies. The reason is that pharmacies have very different arrangements with different prescription plans. When combined together, the cost difference among plans can easily exceed $1,000, a year. It will be many, many thousands of dollars if an expensive medication is not covered by a specific Part D plan.[8]

PREFERRED PHARMACIES AND MAIL ORDER

Prescription plans often use preferred pharmacies and mail order — they should be used whenever possible. When you select a stand-alone prescription drug plan, it is important to input those pharmacies that you frequently use. Only then will you receive an accurate list of the cheapest plans. The same can be said for mail order.

This Happens

Mr. B. has one expensive medication, plus a few generic medications.

The expensive medication has a much

lower copay at one specific pharmacy when compared to other pharmacies. Even though the plan has a deductible that is twice the cost of other competing plans, the overall anticipated drug costs are much lower.

The difference between the first and second most efficient Part D plans is $1,000 a year.

Part D plans have a mail-order option for many prescriptions, and these can reduce out-of-pocket expenses dramatically. That said, some people are not comfortable in receiving prescriptions via mail. Certain medications have a very high "street value," especially in the case of pain-management medications, so special care must be taken in delivery of these sensitive drugs.[9]

CHANGING PLANS

You can change your Part D plan during every Annual Election Period (AEP) without restriction. That means that if your prescriptions change during the year, the best plan may also change. Even if your prescriptions do not change throughout the year, you should still check that your plan is the best for you. The reason? Premiums will change, copays will change, prescription coverage will change for different plans on an annual basis. This means that the plan that fits you best may also change. It may be costly to not check.

IMPORTANT EXTRAS

Prescription Drug Plans Are Reset Annually

The key point here is that prescription drug benefit plans (both Part D and MAPD) are annual contracts, which run from January 1 through December 31. That means all of the terms above are subject to change, every single year. The implication? The anticipated costs can change, even if your medications stay constant from year to year. The difference is notable, resulting in hundreds or thousands of dollars a year, if you stay with your existing plan without choosing efficiently.

Many people choose a stand-alone prescription drug plan (Medicare Part D) and then, simply due to convenience, choose to stay with the same plan. Most do not change, many do not check, and many have never checked to see if they are getting the best possible combination.[10] Given the other advice contained in this book, you can anticipate the reaction to this: bad idea. Even when your prescriptions stay the same, the cost-sharing arrangement can change for the same plan from year to year. That can also result in much higher overall prescription drug costs.

Vaccinations and Flu Shots

Given the headlines in 2019, it is important to note that vaccinations (that is, for shingles) and flu shots are standard in Part D plans; you will be responsible for copays. Many large pharmacy chains provide flu shots without charge if you are covered by a Part D or MAPD plan.

Extra Help Program

Extra Help is a program sponsored by the federal government. It has been known as the Low Income Subsidy (LIS) in the past. If you qualify, the Extra Help program can pay a portion of your Medicare prescription drug costs. The Extra Help program may pay all or part of your monthly Medicare Part D plan premiums and a significant portion of your medication costs.

In order to qualify, you must meet both income and asset tests. To qualify for Extra Help, your resources must be limited to $14,390 for an individual or $28,720 for a married couple living together. Your annual income must be limited to $18,735 for an individual or $25,365 for a married couple living together.[11]

You can apply for the Extra Help program online at https://secure.ssa.gov/i1020/start, by calling Social Security at 1-800-772-1213, and by visiting your local Social Security office.

If you receive Extra Help, then you will also pay either a low or no initial deductible and will not be subject to the coverage gap of Medicare Part D as described in Chapter 5. You do not have the same restriction as others if you qualify for the Extra Help program; that is, you can change plans once per quarter during the first three quarters of 2019, and again during the Annual Election Period.

If you qualify for the Extra Help program, you must be aware that there are number of levels of assistance. In addition, you need to check the letters (don't discard them!) that you receive in order to understand your individual level of assistance, which is subject to change, every year.

Every year, you may receive a letter from the Social Security Administration that will update you on your status. You may be told that you do not qualify for the next year. If this is the case, this is one type of Special Enrollment Period (SEP), and you will be able to adjust your selection of Part D, as well as enroll in a Medicare Advantage Plan or a Medigap plan. You may receive a letter requesting additional information; this is a very important letter (which is one reason to never throw away letters from the CMS), because if you do not answer the letter, then you can lose your access to the Extra Help program entirely.

Money-Saving Tip: Pharmacies Are Important

Choosing Part D plans has become increasingly difficult. The business reality is that Part D (and MAPD) plan carriers have formed alliances with pharmaceutical companies, mail-order delivery providers, and pharmacies. The extent of their collaboration is not the point of this book. However, the implication is very powerful.

Since ownership of Part D and MAPD plans can change, and since these plans have alliances with specific pharmacies or mail-order providers, which pharmacy you use will likely affect your overall prescription cost. This has been true in the past, and it is becoming more extreme.

Anecdotal evidence has proven 2019 to be another extreme year. It used to be the case that a few plans dominated most locations. However, the results vary more wildly, depending on the prescriptions one is prescribed, the tier of each medication, the method of delivery (mail order or retail), and pharmacies.

For example, take latanoprost eyedrops used to treat glaucoma. Prescriptions that are "drops" or "creams" are generally expensive, and different plans handle these prescriptions very differently.

Take Prescription Drug Plan #1. This plan may charge a higher premium, but with no deductible. If so, Latanoprost may not be subject to the high copay under a deductible. Further, pharmacy A may have negotiated a far different price than pharmacy B. The net result is that the most efficient plan for a person that is prescribed latanoprost will result in a multiple hundred-dollar-a-year difference between the first and second most efficient plans available in a particular location.

For people that take the most common generics, the total costs may be the same, assuming that your prescriptions do not change throughout the year. However, what happens if you are prescribed a more expensive medication? Then, on average, the higher priced plan, with no deductible, will result in lower overall costs because the copay structure of higher-premium plans is usually, but not always, superior. You will need to confirm that (and all other facts stated in this book), but it illustrates the point that the lowest monthly premium plan may not be the best choice.

TABLE 3. Medicare Part D Premiums (2020)

Individual	Joint	Monthly Premium
$87,000 or less	$174,000 or less	Plan Premium
$87,000 – $109,000	$174,000 – $218,000	$12.40 + Plan Premium
$109,000 – $136,000	$218,000 -$272,000	$31.90 + Plan Premium
$136,000 – $163,000	$272,000 – $326,000	$51.40 + Plan Premium
$163,000 – $500,000	$326,000 – $750,000	$70.90 + Plan Premium
Greater than $500,000	Greater than $750,000	$77.40 + Plan Premium

Additional amounts ($12.40, $31.90, $51.40, $70.90, and $77.40) will automatically be deducted from your Social Security benefits (if applicable).

Chapter 5
Medicare Advantage

Truths And Myths

Truth: The premiums, deductibles, and co-pays may change every year, so the best overall plan for you can also change.

Truth: Networks must be carefully examined in advance to minimize overall costs.

Myth: Medicare Advantage is always worse than Medigap. This is not true. Medicare Advantage Plans may include important extra benefits (examples: coverage for vision, hearing, wellness, etc.).

The Basics

Medicare Advantage is a Medicare health plan offered by insurance companies that are contracted with Medicare. The insurance company administers all aspects of benefits, billing, and costs. When enrolled in a Medicare Advantage Plan, the insurance company will issue a member card that is to be presented to health-care providers and pharmacies. You will no longer use your traditional red, white, and blue Medicare card (this does not mean that you should discard your traditional Medicare card).

At the end of 2018, Medicare Advantage Plans represented 33 percent of all Medicare beneficiaries, and the popularity of these plans is growing rapidly, a trend that is likely to continue for the immediate future. In many locations in the United States, there may be twenty Medicare Advantage Plans available to choose from, and in some areas, there are as many as sixty separate Medicare Advantage Plans available.

You need to be enrolled in both Medicare Part A and Medicare Part B. You cannot be covered by a Medicare Advantage and Medigap Plan at the same time. At a minimum, Medicare Advantage Plans must cover at least what Original Medicare covers, on average.[1]

There are different types of Medicare Advantage Plans. Medicare Advantage Plans that do not include prescription drug coverage are referred to as MA Plans. Medicare Advantage Plans that include prescription drug benefits are referred to as MAPD (Medicare Advantage Prescription Drug) Plans.

Each year Medicare Advantage Plans are allowed to advertise to Medicare beneficiaries. You are likely to receive many advertisements through the mail regarding Medicare Advantage Plans and will also see television ads. Medicare Advantage Plans available in your area are on the Medicare website at www.medicare.gov, and they may be listed in a physical copy of *Medicare and You.* You can also call Medicare at 1-800-MEDICARE.

TYPES OF MEDICARE ADVANTAGE PLANS

Frequently, the same insurance company will offer clients many Medicare Advantage Plans. This book will refer to the entire set as Medicare Advantage, or MA. This includes plans in which prescription drug coverage is included, known as Medicare

Advantage Prescription Drug Plans (MAPD). Here are the different types of Medicare Advantage Plans:

- HMO (Health Maintenance Organization)
- HMO-POS (HMO Point of Service)
- PPO (Preferred Provider Organization)
- PFFS (Private Fee-for-Service)
- HMO-SNP (Special Needs Plan)
- MSA (Medicare Savings Account)
- MCP (Medicare Cost Plans)
- PACE (Programs of All-Inclusive Care for the Elderly):
- MMP (Medicare-Medicaid Plan)

Each type of Medicare Advantage Plan will differ slightly, and each has some distinctive characteristics.

Health Maintenance Organization (HMO)

You will need to specify a primary-care physician (PCP) who will refer you to specialists as necessary. All providers must be in the network. If you obtain routine medical care from out-of-network medical providers, the HMO may not pay for these services, and you will be responsible for the entire cost. If you use an out-of-network provider, you will be responsible for 100 percent of the cost and those charges will not count toward the health deductible or annual out-of-pocket limit. HMOs can be offered with and without prescription drug benefits.

HMO Point of Service (HMO-POS)

You will need to select a primary-care physician (PCP) who will refer you to specialists as necessary. Deductibles and copays for services provided through the POS contracted network will apply. Coverage for out-of-network services may be provided, but you will have to pay more for these services. Usually the Plan will pay more for out-of-network services if they are referred by the PCP than if you seek these services without a referral.[2]

Preferred Provider Organization (PPO)

You do not need to select a primary-care physician. You can seek medical services from providers outside the network, but with a higher cost-sharing amount. In some cases you may need to pay for out-of-network services and file a claim for reimbursement. Generally, a PPO provider network is larger than a HMO provider network.

Private Fee-for-Service (PFFS)

You can use any Medicare approved provider that accepts the plan's payment and agrees to provide services. The PFFS Plan decides what costs you will be responsible for paying. Some PFFS Plans have a contracted network whose providers agree to always treat you whether or not they have provided service to you in the past. Out-of-network providers may decide not to treat you, even if you have seen them before. A provider has the choice to accept you on a case-by-case basis, except in emergencies. This means that if you go to a doctor for one illness, and you are accepted, that does not guarantee that the same doctor will accept you the next time you attempt to receive services. PFFS Plans might not include prescription drug benefits. PFFS is the only Medicare Advantage Plan in which you can purchase a separate, stand-alone prescription drug plan (Part D).

Special Needs Plan (HMO-SNP)

There are three types of HMO-SNPs.

Chronic Illness (C-SNP)

There are a list of fifteen specific chronic conditions that would qualify you for a C-SNP. There are specific, tailored benefits, formularies, costs, and networks that may apply.

Institutional SNPs (I-SNPs)

The second category applies to when you are resident in a skilled nursing facility.

Dual-Eligible

The third and most predominant type of SNP applies to when you qualify for both Medicare and Medicaid (otherwise known as Dual-Eligible SNP or D-SNP). Under a D-SNP, you must qualify for Medicaid. Within Medicaid, there may be multiple levels of financial assistance, and to qualify for a D-SNP, the carrier will verify your eligibility. These plans have special benefits, beyond the benefits provided by either Medicare or Medicaid alone. A care coordinator may be available at the D-SNP carrier who will be available to assist in arranging transportation, locating helpful social services, and ensuring that prescriptions are being refilled in a timely manner.

Most medical services must be administered by providers in the SNP's network.

Medicare Savings Account (MSA)

MSAs combine a high deductible health plan with a medical savings account. Initially you can use the medical savings account to help pay for health care and then have coverage through a high-deductible insurance plan once you have covered the deductible.

Medicare Cost Plan (MCP)

Medicare Cost Plans are available in certain areas of the country. You can join even if you only have Part B. If you have both Medicare Parts A and B and go to an out-of-network provider, services are covered under Original Medicare, and you will pay the Part A and Part B deductibles and coinsurance. You are not locked in to a Medicare Cost Plan for a specific length of time and can join anytime a Plan is accepting new members and can leave anytime and return to Original Medicare. You can get prescription drug coverage from the Plan, if offered, or you can join any Medicare Prescription Drug Plan.

Programs of All-Inclusive Care for the Elderly (PACE)

PACE is a Medicare and Medicaid Plan that is offered to individuals who can safely live in the community with help but qualify for nursing-home care. To qualify you must be fifty-five years or older, live in the PACE service area, be certified by the state in which you are a resident that you are needing nursing home level of care, and, when you join, be able to live safely in the community with help of PACE services.

Medicare-Medicaid Plan (MMP)

This demonstration plan is designed to provide individuals enrolled in both Medicare and Medicaid with improved healthcare assistance and to improve financial management of Medicare and Medicaid programs. Thirteen states were approved to participate in the MMP demonstration. Currently eleven states are participating.

MEDICARE ADVANTAGE PRESCRIPTION DRUG PLANS

Medicare Advantage Prescription Drug Plans (MAPD) may combine health insurance with prescription drug coverage in one Plan. Some of the different types of Medicare Advantage Plans listed in the previous section can also be an MAPD. For example, an HMO Medicare Advantage Plan might include prescription coverage.

If you have a Medicare Advantage or an MAPD Plan, with one exception you cannot have an additional stand-alone Part D Prescription Drug Plan (PDP). The exception to this is PFFS, in which case you can have a separate PDP. If you elect a Medicare Advantage that does not include prescription benefits and that is ruled as creditable coverage by the Medicare system, then you will have to pay for prescriptions entirely from your own funds. In addition to this, you will be subject to the enrollment penalty at the time that you do enroll in a PDP or MAPD Plan.

In most locations, a limited set of Medicare Advantage Plans are available that do not include prescription drug benefits. TRICARE or Veterans Administration (VA) drug coverage qualifies as creditable coverage. TRICARE, VA, Indian Health Services, Tribal Health Program, and Urban Indian Health Program provide prescription drug benefits. With these plans, you can choose a Medicare Advantage Plan without drug coverage.[3]

ENROLLMENT

Medicare Advantage Initial Enrollment

The Medicare Advantage Initial Coverage Election Period (ICEP) is specific to Medicare Advantage Plans. When you are newly eligible to enroll in MA, you may make an enrollment request during an ICEP. The

ICEP begins three months immediately before your first entitlement to Medicare Part A and Part B and ends on the later of the last day of the month preceding entitlement to both Medicare Part A and Part B or the last day of your Part B initial enrollment period. The last date of the ICEP can differ and can be the source of confusion. It is a bit convoluted and can probably be made clear through an example.

Let's go back to John Smith, born on March 22, 1951.

Case 1: John Smith is turning sixty-five years old on March 22, 2016, and is not working. John is eligible for Medicare Parts A and B on March 1, 2016. Since John has decided to enroll in Part B effective March 1, 2016, the ICEP begins December 1, 2015, and ends June 30, 2016. It is important that these are the same *only* when turning sixty-five years old.

Case 2: John Smith is retiring after he turns sixty-five years of age. Let's say that John Smith is sixty-seven years old and a full-time employee, with health and prescription drug benefits that qualify as creditable coverage, until July 30, 2018, when he retires. He then has eight months to enroll in Medicare Part B. Let's assume he waits until the last possible month and enrolls in Medicare Part B with an effective date of December 1, 2018. That is allowed. John Smith's ICEP would end on November 30, 2018. The latest possible effective date of his Medicare Advantage Plan would be December 1, 2018. He can enroll in any Medicare Advantage Plan with an effective date earlier than December 1, 2018, as long as he is enrolled in both Medicare Part A and Part B.

In Case 1, if he turns sixty-five years old (and only in that instance), John preserves the flexibility to change from Medicare Advantage to Medigap during his twelve-month Trial Period. That will preserve the maximum number of options for him, because he can change his mind and select a Medigap policy without medical underwriting questions. This subtle option does not exist in Case 2. Under Case 2, John would need to pass medical underwriting in order to apply for Medigap, if a Medigap policy is not initially selected.

Under Case 2, John Smith can elect any Medicare Advantage Plan, or can enroll in Medigap without medical underwriting, along with a Part D Plan. However, he does *not* have the twelve-month trial right to switch from Medicare Advantage to Medigap, unless he's within the first six months of enrolling in Part B (irrespective of age).

This is quite a mess, due to the fact that the same terminology (Initial Coverage Election Period, ICEP) is used for both Case 1 and Case 2. The Medicare Advantage twelve-month trial right is powerful, but it can only be used by those first turning sixty-five years old. All is not lost because John may be able to enroll in Medigap due to a different permission (Medigap open enrollment). That said, he would need to be an expert in order to manage the very subtle time frames described here.

The way to resolve all of this for yourself? Enroll in Part B to be effective on your first eligibility date, and carefully decide between Medicare Advantage and Medigap, which will be effective on your Part B effective date. From that point, you will have preserved the maximum flexibility under the rules, under either Case 1 or Case 2.

Medicare Advantage Annual Enrollment Period

After enrolling in Medicare Parts A and B, enrolling in a Medicare Advantage or an

MAPD plan is straightforward. You can enroll in any Medicare Advantage Plan available in your geographical location during the Annual Election Period (AEP). Every year, the AEP runs from October 15 through December 7, a period of seven weeks.

During the AEP, you can change your mind as many times as you would like. The last plan that you elect based on the date on your enrollment forms will be the Plan that is in effect on the following January 1.

If you cancel a Medigap policy in order to enroll in Medicare Advantage, you must separately cancel the Medigap carrier. The cancellation of the old Medigap policy is not automatic, and only the Medigap policyholder has the authority to cancel. You can contact the customer service department at the Medigap carrier, and it will provide specific instructions on how to cancel.

Medicare Advantage Twelve-Month Trial Right

If you enroll in a Medicare Advantage Plan before the date that you are first eligible for Medicare Part A and Part B at the age of sixty-five, then you can cancel at any time during your first twelve months under that

Plan and return to Original Medicare. You can then enroll in a Medigap Plan (along with a stand-alone prescription Plan, Medicare Part D) or simply stay with Original Medicare. You will not be subject to medical underwriting in this instance.

OPEN ENROLLMENT PERIOD

The Medicare Advantage Disenrollment Period no longer exists, beginning in 2019. Instead, a *new* enrollment period will run between January 1 and March 31, 2019, called the Open Enrollment Period. Here is what you can and cannot do:

- You can change to another Medicare Advantage Plan with or without drug coverage, only if you are already a Medicare Advantage member. You can make this change once during the Open Enrollment Period. This can be valuable for those that want to add prescription coverage under Medicare Advantage. There are reasons that you may want to use this time period to change among Medicare Advantage Plans. For example, you may discover that the in-network providers have changed. Or, you may discover that a different carrier offers additional benefits that suit your requirements.

- You can disenroll from your Medicare Advantage Plan, return to Original Medicare, and enroll in a Prescription Drug Plan. This will allow you to separately choose a Medicare Part D plan. Note that this does not guarantee acceptance into Medigap. Medigap underwriting rules are still in full effect.[4] This means that if you want to use this period to switch from Medicare Advantage to Medigap you can, but it is very important to first secure acceptance into Medigap. Not doing so could result in having Part A, Part B, and Part D, but no other coverage. That would leave you completely responsible for the Part A inpatient hospital deductible, the Part A copays, the Part B deductible, and the 20 percent coinsurance not paid by Medicare Part B.
- If you enrolled in a Medicare Advantage Plan during your Initial Enrollment Period, you can change to another Medicare Advantage Plan (with or without drug coverage) or go back to Original Medicare (with or without drug coverage) within the first three months you have Medicare.

- You can enroll in Original Medicare (Part A and Part B) if you have not correctly enrolled in Medicare when you were first eligible. Your effective date will not be until July 1 of that year.
- You cannot be a new enrollee in a Medicare Advantage Plan. This period is only open to those that are already Medicare Advantage members.
- You cannot enroll in a Prescription Drug Plan if you are in Original Medicare.
- You cannot change among Medicare Part D plans.
- You cannot switch from Medigap to Medicare Advantage.

Special Enrollment Periods (SEPs)

Medicare allows people that have special situations to be able to elect a Medicare Advantage Plan outside the Annual Election Period. Depending on the reason for the Special Enrollment Period, an individual may:

- Discontinue an enrollment in an MA Plan and enroll in Original Medicare.
- Switch from Original Medicare to an MA Plan.

- Switch from one MA Plan to another MA Plan.

Here is a list of twelve such situations. There are more than this, and additional ones can be added by the CMS with little advance notice:

1. Change in residence: If you have moved your permanent residence outside the service area of your current MA Plan or if new Medicare Plans or Prescription Drug Plans are available. If you move from outside the US, where you were living permanently, then you qualify. Individuals not eligible for MA due to incarceration who have been released may enroll through the SEP.
2. Medicaid Status Change: If your Medicaid status changes, then you qualify.
3. Low Income Subsidy (Extra Help): If you are eligible for the Low Income Subsidy (Extra Help), then you can change without restriction at any time during the calendar year, once per quarter for the first three quarters in a year. You can additionally change plans during the Annual Election

Period.

4. Skilled Nursing Facility Care: If you are moving in or out of a skilled nursing care facility, then you qualify.
5. PACE (Program of All-Inclusive Care for the Elderly): If you leave a PACE program, then you qualify. PACE is only available in selected states.
6. Loss of Creditable Coverage: If your prescription drug benefits are ruled to no longer be creditable coverage, then you qualify. "Creditable coverage" is defined in the Glossary.
7. Employer-Sponsored Plan Change: If you are losing your coverage from an employer-sponsored benefit plan, then you qualify.
8. Pharmacy Assistance Program: If you are entering a Qualified State Pharmaceutical Assistance Program (SPAP) or if you have lost your eligibility, then you qualify.
9. Other Prescription Drug Assistance: If you no longer qualify for other prescription drug assistance that you have been receiving, then you qualify for an SEP.
10. Medicare Advantage Plan Cancellation: If your Medicare Advantage Plan is no longer in existence, then you

qualify (you must elect this SEP only between December 8 and the end of February of the following year).

11. Five-Star Plan: If you want to switch to a Medicare Advantage Plan that is rated as "five star" by the CMS, then you qualify, without calendar restriction. You can switch to a five-star plan only once during a calendar year.
12. Special Circumstances: There can be special circumstances that occur. For example, if your location has been declared a disaster area by a governmental party (FEMA or your governor) or if the HHS has declared a public health emergency, then the CMS may grant a limited Special Enrollment Period.

A general rule of thumb is that if you qualify for an SEP, then you have two months (sixty-three days) from the date that you begin an SEP to adopt a new plan, whether that is another Medicare Advantage Plan or a new Medicare Part D plan, regardless of the reasons listed here.[5]

Using Medicare Plan Finder

Once you have decided to enroll in a Medicare Advantage or Medicare Advantage Prescription Drug Plan, then the question is, what is the best plan for you? The answer will require some work on your part. You may request the assistance of an expert or a professional. You can do it yourself by going to www.medicare.gov. Here are the steps to take:

1. Click "Find Health & Drug Plans."
2. Choose "Continue without logging in." It is important to not login because doing so will allow all of your personal, private Medicare information to be viewed on your computer.
3. Choose "View plans. I know what type of plan I want."
4. Choose "Medicare Advantage Plan."
5. Enter your zip code and choose the correct county of residence.
6. Choose "no" under "Do you have a Medicare number?" While you can choose "yes," remember that this means you will be logging in, and your private, personal information, including claims history, will be viewable.

7. Enter your date of birth.
8. Answer "Do you get help with your costs from one of these programs?" It is an important step, so choose the correct option. The premiums may vary if you receive extra help. Choose "Next."
9. "Do you want to see your drug costs when you compare plans?" Choose "Yes."
10. "How do you normally fill your prescriptions?" Choose "Both." Again, this is important because you are attempting to identify the lowest-cost drug coverage. It is not necessarily the case that mail order is the least expensive.
11. Enter your prescription drugs. It is very important to enter the generic drug name, if you are using a generic form. Once completed, choose "Done."
12. Choose pharmacies from the list. When complete, choose "Done."
13. You will see a list of Medicare Advantage plans available in your zip code.
14. Find "Sort plans by," and choose "Lowest drug cost." The results will be sorted in order of lowest prescription drug costs, not including premium.[6]

There are important limitations to the report. First, the out-of-pocket costs for health-care services are not compared on this report. This means that if you require hospitalization, diagnostic services, specialist office visits, etc., you cannot readily compare plans. Second, the combination of physicians and hospitals is not confirmed using the Medicare Plan Finder. There is no shortcut; you will need to examine this yourself. In every case, insurance carriers have websites where you can review whether the physician/hospital accepts the specific Medicare Advantage Plan.[7]

How to Compare Medicare Advantage Plans

The improvements in Medicare Advantage since the first edition of *Maximize Your Medicare* in 2013 have been dramatic. Networks have expanded, access to specialists can occur with referral, prescription drug benefits can exceed stand-alone Part D Plans, and health and prescription deductibles can be as low as $0.

If anything, this has made it more difficult to tell exactly which Medicare Advantage Plan is best. Here's the starting point we use with our clients nationwide.

Deductible

Under Medicare Advantage, there are separate health and prescription drug deductibles. The stunning development in 2019 is the continued evidence of lower health and drug deductibles among Medicare Advantage Plans. There are now Medicare Advantage Plans with health deductibles of $0 and plans with drug deductibles that are dramatically lower than the federal standard of $435. This is very valuable to the millions of people who live on a fixed, monthly income because it allows people to plan their monthly spending budgets carefully, especially at the beginning of the year.

Out-of-Pocket Costs

Each Medicare Advantage Plan will have its own cost-sharing arrangements, a plan-specific set of terms and conditions that can require a certain schedule of payments for office visits (other than the preventative-care checkup, which is complimentary under the Affordable Care Act), hospital stays, skilled nursing care facilities, durable medical equipment, and everything else under Medicare Part A and Part B. The deductible, coinsurance, and copayment amounts are fully detailed in your "Summary of Benefits" guide and Explanation of

Benefits (EOB), and the coverage that you receive in a Medicare Advantage or MAPD must be at least as good as the benefits that you receive under Original Medicare, on average.

Part B Premium Rebate

For enrollees in certain Medicare Advantage Plans, a portion of the Part B premium ($135.50 a month for new enrollees) can be rebated, in the form of a higher Social Security benefit. Those who receive government assistance for Part B premiums, resulting from Medicaid payments, are not eligible.

Prescriptions

As noted earlier, the improvement to prescription drug benefits has been dramatic and yet, it will very much depend on your specific prescriptions. It is entirely the case that the selection of Medicare Advantage Plan will depend on the overall estimated cost of prescriptions. This holds especially true, since the remainder of factors in this section are very competitive, that there can be virtually no difference. However, the same cannot be said about prescription drug benefits, and that means that this is an area that can determine which Medicare

Advantage Plan is best.

Hospital Stay Copay

There are two ways that most Medicare Advantage Plans offer cost-sharing if you are admitted to the hospital. You should choose the copay that is a given cost per stay, and not the deductible that charges per day. Why? Simply put, you usually get admitted to a hospital for longer than a single night. Therefore, when you multiply the per-day copay times the number of days, that is usually more than the copay that is charged by those plans that charge on a per-stay basis. All else equal, the premium will, on average, be slightly higher, but the fact is that if you stay at a hospital for multiple days, then you will save money by choosing a Medicare Advantage Plan that charges you per stay, and not on a per-day basis.

Office Visits

If there is a plan that does not distinguish between your family physician and a specialist, then that should be chosen, since an office visit to a specialist may be substantially more expensive than an office visit to your primary-care physician.

Extra Benefits

Many Medicare Advantage Plans include discounts on dental and vision, weight-loss, and smoking-cessation programs. Complimentary health club memberships, or discounts for health club memberships, are widely found. Extensive, specialized dental work, such as implants or treatment of gum disease, are generally not covered by these extra benefits. In fact, as many know, serious dental work is usually uncovered by any type of dental insurance, and the maximum benefit is limited. In 2018, the rules for the types of extra benefits allowed under Medicare Advantage have been relaxed. This means that there are now benefits for items like in-home shower bars. It is complicated, but this particular area has the potential to entirely change the health insurance landscape, because if those benefits can be proven to lower health-care costs overall, they may be offered as additional benefits to Medicare Advantage members.

MEDICARE ADVANTAGE HAS IMPROVED

Since the first edition of *Maximize Your Medicare* in 2013, the most dramatic change to Medicare has been the improvement in Medicare Advantage. Specifically, prescription drug coverage within Medicare Advantage Plans has been greatly improved. It is entirely possible that the prescription drug costs within Medicare Advantage are superior to benefits provided by stand-alone prescription drug Plans (Part D).

This Happens
An insulin-dependent diabetic has multiple medications and is enrolled in Medigap along with Part D. Copays of medications put the diabetic into the Part D coverage gap. However, he discovers a Medicare Advantage Prescription Drug Plan in which the specific insulin he uses is categorized as a Tier 2 generic. The copay for that generic: $0.

Medicare Advantage May Be Superior to Medigap

The pressure on the Medicare system has resulted in the elimination of certain treatments and consultations, or limited the inclusion of others. For example, one type of service being limited is the consultation with certain specialists. The implication here is that Medigap will not cover these treatments or consultations if Original Medicare does not cover them. However, certain Medicare Advantage Plans may provide these valuable benefits.

Notably, observation status has already been addressed by certain Medicare Advantage Plans. You can recall Chapter 2, where the principle of "Observation Status" is addressed. Under Original Medicare, an inpatient status is required and that stay must be for three days in order to receive skilled nursing care benefits under Medicare Part A. However, some carriers have altered this in a very positive way, because beneficiaries of certain Medicare Advantage Plans can receive skilled nursing care benefits without a three-day inpatient hospital stay.

Consumers Must Understand Networks

The most important aspect of Medicare Advantage (MA) coverage is the concept of network. Most people have experienced a health-care network of some sort, whether in the form of your employer's group health insurance Plan or private health insurance. For Medicare Advantage, a similar concept applies. When you receive services from providers inside the network, cost-sharing is reasonable. Outside the network, however, cost-sharing greatly increases the out-of-pocket deductibles, copays, and annual out-of-pocket maximums. That is why it is important to check the physicians that you visit, as well as those that you might be reasonably expected to visit.

Doctors might accept a particular Medicare Advantage Plan; do not assume that your doctor will accept your Medicare Advantage Plan, even if he/she accepted your employer's plan in the past, and even if he/she accepted insurance from the same carrier before you were under Medicare. Medicare networks can be entirely separate, and you need to check this for yourself (or with a professional's assistance).[8]

HMOs, in particular, deserve very specific examination, because in many cases, you can only go to a specialist after receiving a referral from your primary-care physician (PCP). That specialist must also belong to the network.

For PPOs, out-of-network providers will accept any Medicare Advantage Plan, but you will be charged a different amount for services received. In addition, the annual out-of-pocket maximum is notably higher if you use out-of-network providers.

One thing that you must keep in mind is that if you travel on vacation and you require medical attention, then the provider you visit might not be inside the network. It is important to note that certain, nationally prominent insurance companies will allow much wider access of doctors, hospitals, and clinics to be "in network." This is one area that Medicare Advantage carriers have improved. While the improvement in networks does not completely eliminate your responsibility to double-check, and there are challenges that remain, the situation has improved greatly.

Networks can change, midyear, without notice. There are a number of cases when a hospital, physician, or other health-care provider has been added to a carrier's network, and the opposite can be true. This can be due to a wide variety of reasons, all beyond the consumer's control. Unfortunately, there is no easy solution to this problem. While the number of instances of this occurring is limited, it does happen.

SURPRISE MEDICAL BILLS

If you are in a hospital, you may require some diagnostic services, or a specialist may be called in order to provide additional services. You may receive a bill for these services, and, depending on the type of Medicare Advantage Plan that you have, you may receive a nasty surprise.

If the lab or specialist is out of network, then your out-of-pocket expenses may either be higher than expected, or you may be responsible for 100 percent of the costs.

PPO

In this example, the health-care provider can be in-network, which would result in the lowest copay to you. Or, the health-care provider can be out-of-network, and you would be responsible for a higher copay amount. In addition, the annual out-of-pocket maximum will likely be higher for you, because there is a higher out-of-pocket maximum limit when you use both in-network and out-of-network providers.

HMO

In this example, you may be responsible for 100 percent of the costs, if the lab or physician is not in-network. This creates an unexpected, unwelcome surprise, because you may have not been informed of this fact in advance.

These types of situations have received a great deal of public attention. There is a movement and proposed legislation to reduce or eliminate this situation. As of this writing, surprise medical bills can still occur when you receive health-care services from a person or location that you did not realize was out of network.

Out-of-Pocket Maximum Limit

Every Medicare Advantage Plan must have an annual out-of-pocket limit (MOOP). This is critical, because, as mentioned in Chapters 2 and 3, Original Medicare Part A and Part B have no annual out-of-pocket limit. A Medicare Advantage Plan puts a cap on your out-of-pocket health-care costs, and there are many plans that have no additional premium.

The annual out-of-pocket limits can differ under PPOs, when you use a combination of in-network and out-of-network providers. In every case, when you use a combination of in-network and out-of-network providers, the out-of-pocket maximum limit is much higher. (Sometimes this cannot be avoided; see "Surprise Medical Bills" in this chapter.) Nevertheless, this is still a superior financial outcome compared to an HMO, when you would be fully responsible for all costs if a provider was not in network.

The annual out-of-pocket cost calculation does not include amounts charged above the Medicare allowed charge. The Medicare allowed charge has been described in Chapter 3. Certain Medicare Advantage Plans address this by disallowing providers from charging any additional amounts to Medicare Advantage beneficiaries.

Annual Notice of Change (ANOC)

Every year, both Medicare Advantage Plans and stand-alone prescription plan (Part D) beneficiaries will begin to receive an Annual Notice of Change (ANOC), a regulatory requirement mandated by the CMS. The ANOC will contain detailed information regarding coverage you have received in the current year and will display how it will change in the following year. For example, the ANOC will display changes in premiums, deductibles, and copays, which may vary from year to year, depending on the services that you receive.

It cannot be overstated: Beneficiaries should read these ANOCs when received. Too often, beneficiaries discard this document and learn, after the fact, that their out-of-pocket costs change at a time they least expect. A very important feature about all Medicare Advantage and Medicare Part D Plans is that they are annual contracts. Plans are approved by the CMS on an annual basis and can be greatly affected by a large number of factors.

Last (and not least), Medicare Advantage Plans and Part D Plans are actively competing against one another. The result is that the terms and conditions of your Medicare Advantage or Medicare Part D are likely to change, and those changes can affect the cost of the coverage and services you receive.

MEDICARE AND MEDICAID

A special type of D-SNP (Dual Special Needs Plan) is for those that are enrolled in both Medicaid and Medicare, called "Dual Eligible." Medicaid eligibility is determined by the state of residence and is complicated, since each state has its own separate rules.

This subset of Medicare Advantage Plans frequently provides benefits beyond the benefits provided by both Medicare and Medicaid. For example, there can be additional dental, hearing, vision, and transportation benefits. In addition, there can be specific care-management personnel who will be available to help coordinate timely refills of prescriptions and assist with access to community services.

In most instances, there is no premium, and dual eligibles are able to switch among D-SNPs once per quarter, and once during the Annual Election Period, which runs from October 15 through December 7. This right to change among plans exists for

Medicaid beneficiaries, because all Medicaid beneficiaries are enrolled in the federal Extra Help program.

Extra Help and Medicare Advantage

If you receive Extra Help, which is the federal assistance program to help pay for prescription drug benefits, then your Extra Help assistance might affect the published Medicare Advantage premium. Every year, the allocation toward your Medicare Advantage premium is subject to change. The results will differ from plan to plan, from year to year. The implication is very powerful.

Let's take a simple example:

MAPD Plan 1, a PPO, premium is $60.
MAPD Plan 2, an HMO, premium is $35.
MAPD Plan 1, the PPO, with Extra Help benefits, premium is $30.
MAPD Plan 2, an HMO, with Extra Help benefits, premium is $35.

You can see that MAPD Plan 2 has intentionally not used your Extra Help benefits toward a lowering of the premium. However, MAPD Plan 1 has allocated $30 a month toward lowering the premium. Perhaps you preferred MAPD Plan 1, but found it too expensive. After examining this example, you can see that you may choose MAPD Plan 1 with Extra Help at a lower premium than MAPD 2.

When researching plans on the Medicare Plan Finder (www.medicare.gov), be sure to select "I Applied for and Got Extra Help from Social Security." This will create a different set of estimates and reports than would have been otherwise created.

Snowbirds

A "snowbird" (a person who goes to warm-weather locations during the winter) may vacation for extended periods of time. However, when that person goes to his or her physician in Arizona (or Florida, etc.), the physician may not belong to the network, and the out-of-network cost-sharing arrangement would apply. The price differential can be so great that it would have justified more comprehensive coverage via another selection.

Not all insurance companies are equal, of course. Some are far more dominant in particular states, or in a particular location. Others are more national in scope and scale. You should think carefully if you are going to choose a Medicare Advantage Plan and check your medical providers in advance to minimize your out-of-pocket costs. Most of the time, the insurance companies have online directories, so you can search for your providers, or you can ask your insurance representative/agent for assistance.

In addition, you will be faced with a very complicated situation with respect to annual out-of-pocket maximums if you are enrolled in a Medicare Advantage Plan. The reason this occurs is because some of your expenses will be in-network, and other will be out-of-network. You will need to keep track of your visits, and the charges, in order to reconcile the statement of benefits that you receive from the insurance company that issued your Medicare Advantage Plan. That alone is the source of great confusion because then you will basically be forced to verify your Medicare Advantage's records by comparing them to bills received.

Foreign Travel

Health benefits when travelling outside the United States are not included in Original Medicare. However, many Medicare Advantage Plans have added health benefits for those that are travelling to foreign countries on vacation. Every Medicare Advantage

Plan can have a different set of terms and conditions; you will need to check your Explanation of Benefits (EOB).

CHAPTER 6
MEDIGAP

TRUTHS AND MYTHS

Myth: Medigap premiums increase at the random choice of the carrier. This is not correct because there are regulations that require carriers to spend at least 80 percent of premiums on claims, and if they do not, the balance is refunded to you.

Truth: Medigap benefits do not change from year to year. Premiums are likely to increase with age.

Truth: Plan C, Plan F, and High-Deductible Plan F are not available to you as a new applicant, beginning January 1, 2020, unless your Medicare Part A and Part B coverage dates are both prior to January 1, 2020. Depending on the carrier, you may be able to change your existing Medigap Plan to Plans C, F, and High-Deductible F, but that will depend on the carrier and your state.

Truth: Acceptance into Medigap, when turning sixty-five years old, is unrestricted and you will receive the best possible premium. However, enrolling in Medigap later can be based on your health at the time that you apply. At that time, your application can be denied at the discretion of the insurance carrier.

Medigap, Medicare Supplements, and Medicare Supplemental are three different terms that can be found, but they all describe the same set of plans. For the purposes of this book, the term Medigap will be used.[1] There are eleven Medigap plans, with letters A through N (some plans are no longer available). These plans are standardized — the coverage of Medigap Plan A, and all other plans, is the same regardless of the name of the insurance carrier.

This chapter will describe the terms and conditions of those plans, as well as the enrollment timeline. The conclusion will be that Medigap plans, along with a standalone prescription drug plan (PDP), may be better for you than any other configuration that exists in the market, due to features overwhelmingly in the policyowner's favor. It will be up to the consumer to determine if the higher premiums are worth it when compared to Medicare Advantage.

MEDIGAP ENROLLMENT

Medigap Open Enrollment Timing

The Medigap open enrollment period is not the same as the Medicare Initial Enrollment Period. The Medigap open enrollment period begins on the first day of the month that you become eligible for Medicare Part B, and it lasts for six months.[2]

Depending on the state, you can apply prior to the beginning of the Medigap open enrollment period. Remember John Smith, born in March, 1951? March 1, 2016 is the regulated beginning of John Smith's Medigap open enrollment period, but he will very likely be able to apply in advance. That will depend on the state and/or insurance company, but it is usually the case. An easy rule of thumb is that when the Medicare Initial Coverage Election Period (IEP) begins, you can usually sign up for Medigap. We will see other important situations when there are federal regulations, but carriers exceed these minimum standards.

John Smith turns sixty-five on March 22, 2016. The way that Medigap open enrollment period strictly works is that his open enrollment period begins on March 1, 2016 and lasts through August 31, 2016.

Medigap Open Enrollment Rights

During the Medigap open enrollment period, your application will be approved, and you can choose any Medigap plan available by any insurance company that offers Medigap in your geographical location. During the Medigap open enrollment period, insurance companies cannot deny you coverage, nor can they charge you a higher price based on your medical situation. While insurance companies are obligated to accept you, however, they can charge different prices based on your biological sex. It is reasonable to anticipate that this will continue.

Guaranteed Issue (Medicare Protections)

Guaranteed Issue is slightly different than Medigap open enrollment. You will be able to select a subset of Medigap plans if you are entitled to a Special Enrollment Period (SEP), as described in Chapter 5. This is difficult because the different Guaranteed Issue rules allow you to enroll in a different set of Medigap plans. Guaranteed Issue allows you to enroll in Plans A, B, G, K, and L.

In some cases, you can choose any Medigap plan available in your location due to state-specific regulations. In other cases, only a subset of Medigap plans is available. Finally, there are state-specific rules that may grant you additional rights to enroll in Medigap without medical underwriting.

Carriers cannot deny your application in these instances, according to Guaranteed Issue rules for Medigap:[3]

- You are in a Medicare Advantage Plan, and your plan is leaving Medicare or stops giving care in your area, or you move out of the plan's service area.
- You have Original Medicare and an employer group health plan (including retiree or COBRA coverage) or union coverage that pays after Medicare pays, and that plan is ending.
- You have Original Medicare and a Medicare SELECT policy. You move out of the Medicare SELECT policy's service area.
- (Trial Right) You joined a Medicare Advantage Plan or Programs of All-inclusive Care for the Elderly (PACE) when you were first eligible for Medicare Part A at sixty-five, and within the first year of joining, you decide you want to switch to Original Medicare.

- (Trial Right) You dropped a Medigap policy to join a Medicare Advantage Plan (or to switch to a Medicare SELECT policy) for the first time; you have been in the plan less than a year, and you want to switch back.[4]
- Your Medigap insurance company goes bankrupt, and you lose your coverage, or your Medigap policy coverage otherwise ends through no fault of your own.
- You leave a Medicare Advantage Plan or drop a Medigap policy because the company hasn't followed the rules, or it misled you.
- If you qualify under these circumstances, then you will have sixty-three days to apply for Medicare. In addition to the ability to purchase a Medigap policy, the SEP will allow you to enroll in a stand-alone prescription drug plan (PDP/Medicare Part D).

Guaranteed Acceptance

While Medigap open enrollment and special enrollment periods are clear, and protected by federal regulations, that is not the full story. The practical reality is that carriers or states have widened the acceptance rules into Medigap, under certain conditions.[5]

The bottom line is that if you believe that Medigap is best, then these expanded pathways do exist.

The term being used by carriers is "guaranteed acceptance." It is very important to note that this is not exactly the same thing as Guaranteed Issue when applying for Medigap. What this means is that your Medigap application will be accepted under certain conditions, in addition to the Guaranteed Issue regulations, which are federally mandated. Again, either the state or the carrier can elect to grant these wider, more lenient standards.[6]

Let's take an example. Under Guaranteed Issue, a person's retiree health plan must end, and the applicant would be "forced out," involuntarily ejected from the soon-to-be nonexistent retiree health benefits plan. In that case, the applicant would be allowed to enroll in any Medigap under Guaranteed Issue ("Medigap Protections"). However, if a person wants to *voluntarily* end his retiree health benefits plan and enroll in Medigap, then he would be required to apply, and the application would be subject to medical underwriting. However, if the applicant lives in a location where guaranteed acceptance exists, and if he can locate the carrier that offers Medigap, then it may be entirely possible that his application would be accepted without medical underwriting. In this example, the applicant could voluntarily elect to cancel retiree health benefits and enroll in a Medigap policy without medical underwriting.

Simplified Underwriting

Depending on the carrier, an applicant may be subject to much more lenient medical underwriting questions than is normally the case. This means that while "normal" underwriting may have resulted in rejection, carriers may not even ask the "normal" questions but far fewer questions, which will allow certain applicants to be accepted when they would otherwise have been rejected.[7]

Medigap Coverage

Medigap coverage is very simple and straightforward. Medigap will cover all costs associated with Part A.[8] You, the policyholder, will be responsible for the Part B deductible, as stated in Chapter 3. Once you have met the Part B deductible, and the CMS possesses records that you have met it, then Medigap will cover all of the 20 percent that Part B does not cover. For policyholders of Plan G, Medigap will cover the Part B Excess as well.

Table 4 at the end of this chapter provides the standardized guide. The name of the carrier does not matter: every "Plan X" is identical to each other. Further, the terms and conditions of coverage, as summarized in Table 4, do not change over time. There are no exceptions to this.

MEDIGAP AND MEDICARE PART A

You can see in Table 4 that every Medigap plan will pay, either in full or in part, the Part A deductible when you are admitted on an inpatient basis to a hospital. That makes every Medigap plan vastly better than Original Medicare. You may remember from Chapter 2 (on Medicare Part A) that the deductible for hospital admission is $1,408 per benefit period. In all plans except Plan K, Plan L, and High-Deductible Plan F, the entire deductible is paid. This compares very favorably with Original Medicare and Medicare Advantage Plans.

In addition, all Medigap plans will cover at least 50 percent of the coinsurance amount ($176) from days twenty-one to one hundred in a skilled nursing care facility. For example, if you have a joint replacement surgery and you enter a rehabilitation center for a period longer than expected, your Medigap plan will cover at least 50 percent of the $176 a day that the Medicare system does not cover. Under most Medigap plans, the Medigap plan will cover the entire $176 per day.[9]

Beyond the one-hundredth day, you are responsible for 100 percent of all costs at a skilled nursing facility. There are no plans (Medigap or Medicare Advantage) that provide benefits beyond the one-hundredth day.

MEDIGAP AND MEDICARE PART B

With respect to Medicare Part B, you can see again by Table 4 that many of the Medigap plans cover most, if not all, costs not covered by Medicare Part B. In most cases, you are responsible for the Part B deductible, which must be paid (and reconciled at the CMS) before Medigap benefits are received.[10]

Coinsurance that accompanies Medicare Part B is paid in full by all Medigap plans except K and L, in which Medigap pays 50 percent (or 75 percent for Plan L) of the 20 percent that Original Medicare Part B does not pay. For all other plans (except for High-Deductible Plan F, which is described later in this chapter), a Medigap policy pays for the entire 20 percent that is not covered by Medicare Part B.

One specific Medigap plan (Plan N) charges a fee per office visit. You can see it's a maximum of $20 for most office visits. To be clear, the annual preventative care examination is still free, in accordance with the Affordable Care Act (ACA). Under Plan N, it is $50 per visit to an emergency room.[11]

Since Plans C and F are not available to new Medicare beneficiaries, unless your Part A and Part B coverage dates are both prior to January 1, 2020, Plan G is the single Medigap plan that will cover Part B excess charges, described in Chapter 3.

Exception: Medicare SELECT

In some states, you may be able to buy another type of Medigap policy called Medicare SELECT. SELECT plans provide coverage using the same terms as other Medigap policies, but they may require you to use certain health-care providers. The result is that the premium may be less than standard Medigap plans. You can be charged more if you receive services that are not part of a prespecified list.

Medicare SELECT premiums will be lower than Medigap plans, all else equal. However, SELECT plans do introduce networks, which eliminates a major advantage of Medigap. You should carefully compare whether the premium savings are worth the network limitation. In 2018, there were multiple instances where lists of network participants in Medicare SELECT changed within the calendar year.

The bottom line is that unless the cost savings is worth choosing a Medicare SELECT plan instead of a standardized Medigap plan, the standardized Medigap plan is superior because all health-care providers that accept Medicare (the red, white, and blue card) will accept your Medigap card.

PREMIUMS

There are a few different ways that Medigap premiums are determined. However, your specific claims do not affect your specific premiums in the future. That is not the way that insurance normally works; the premiums depend on the population of policyholders at your carrier, as determined by the carrier.[12]

Attained-Age vs. Issue-Age vs. Community

There are three different pricing mechanisms for Medigap policies: attained age, issue age, and community. In reality, they are quite straightforward to understand. The availability of the different types of plans varies depending on your state. This book will address the three types in order of popularity.

Attained age assigns a premium when you apply and adjusts over time. This is the dominant method that you will find available in most locations. Attained age has a separate price depending upon your actual age at the time you apply.

Let's revisit John Smith, who becomes eligible on March 1, 2016. He will be offered a price for a sixty-five-year-old male. Depending upon the insurance company, the premium may stay constant for a prestated period. Insurance companies have the right to change premiums as long as they can prove that claims are 80 percent of the premiums, minus administrative and other various charges. This is called the Medical Loss Ratio (MLR). The important fact is that when John turns sixty-six, he can be charged a different premium. He cannot be charged a different premium based on his individual claims (a frequently asked question by many).

Under attained age, you can experience multiple increases in a year. How? Let's say you turned sixty-five in May and were offered a twelve-month premium guarantee.

When you turn sixty-six, your premium will be that of a sixty-six-year-old. If the carrier changes its overall rates in August, then you could be charged a new twelve-month premium in August. That is entirely possible.

Community has a single price regardless of age. It does not differ whether you are sixty-five or eighty. This has an obvious advantage, which is that as you get older, it may make sense to have a community-based Medigap policy, if you are permitted to do so. That said, the premium of a community policy should be higher than the attained-age policy for the same person who is new to Medicare. The other issue to consider is that even though the price is not different if you are sixty-five or eighty, the price for the entire community of policyholders may increase.

Issue-age policies are priced when you first purchase the plan, and the price does not change. Like community policies, issue-age policies have a price that is initially higher than the more popular attained-age policy.

It is almost impossible to predict which type of pricing will work out best over the long run. The simple logic is that it is very difficult to outguess the virtually unlimited computing power available to insurance companies. Recall from the Introduction to this book that these are financial contracts; the premiums are determined by commercial competition and statistics, not politics or personal opinion.

ADVANTAGES OF MEDIGAP

When considering whether Medigap is best, notice that there are characteristics that exist in all Medigap policies.[13]

Base Case: Medigap Is Superior

If you read the Introduction to this book, you can remember that the main objective here is for you to avoid catastrophic financial losses.[14] Some events, like a hurricane, cannot be anticipated. Of course, no one wants to get ill. However, if illness occurs, as is more likely when you age, then financial costs can add up and cost you a significant portion of your retirement savings. No one can avoid the natural aging process and the increased likelihood of getting ill that accompanies the passage of time.

If you enter into a situation when the Part A deductible or coinsurance is due, then Medigap can save you money, and there is no concept of network, as mentioned earlier. For those that don't like the guesswork of calculating how much you will owe when you receive medical services from your physician, Medigap provides clarity and consistency. The benefits provided by your Medigap policy next year will be calculated the same way it is calculated this year.

Standardization and Grandfathering

Two features of Medigap make it extraordinarily stable. Let's call these features standardization and grandfathering. Through standardization, the coverage for all Plan Ns is the same, regardless of insurance company. That makes it easier for medical-provider administrators/billing personnel to understand. The idea of language that changes from company to company, odd definitions that change, and hidden language simply does not exist.

The second and potentially more important reason that a Medigap policy is superior to any other policy is because of the grandfathering characteristic. This is known as "Guaranteed Renewable." As long as you continue to pay premiums, the policy remains in effect as it was originally written, unless it is changed by the CMS. The only party that can cancel your policy is you. As long as you continue to pay the premium, renewal is a certainty, with no action required.

In the past, the Medicare system had discontinued plans but allowed persons who were originally enrolled in that plan to remain. That is very important, largely because we may anticipate, or reasonably predict, that the Medicare system will change in the future. As you may have read, doomsday predictions suggest that the Medicare system will be insolvent as soon as 2026. For the record, this isn't a plausible scenario (the most influential voting bloc is over fifty years old). However, it is entirely possible, if not probable, that certain plans may be discontinued in the future.

No Network

Unlike Medicare Advantage Plans, Medigap has no concept of network. If your medical doctor or medical provider accepts Original Medicare, he or she will accept your Medigap coverage. Sometimes, you will get pushback from a secretary or billing coordinator, who asks you what Medigap plan you may have. The question is actually quite annoying for a billing professional to ask, because it actually is irrelevant. It isn't even a question that the billing coordinator should be asking. At the risk of being repetitive, if a doctor or medical provider accepts Medicare, they are required to accept your Medigap policy, regardless of location.

Right to Switch

The base case is that you can easily switch from Medigap to Medicare Advantage, but you may not be able to switch easily from Medicare Advantage to Medigap. You can always cancel Medigap and select a Medicare Advantage Plan during the Annual Election Period. The same cannot be said in reverse. After the Medigap open enrollment period expires, an insurance company can deny your application, based on its rights to ask medical underwriting questions.[15]

Put simply, let's say there are two policies. One policy allows you to switch freely; let's call it Contract A. One does not; let's call it Contract B. If everything else were equal, Contract A would be worth more than Contract B. You don't need to know anything about insurance to understand this concept. If everything else were equal, Medigap (Contract A) is more expensive than Medicare Advantage (Contract B). Of course, everything is not equal: Medigap usually costs more than a Medicare Advantage Plan. The practical reality is that a portion of the cost difference you pay is for the right to be able to change later. For further analysis, see the "Experts' Addendum."

This Happens

A sixty-seven-year-old is informed that his retiree health insurance plan is going to be canceled by his employer. He faces two issues. First, he is protected by Guaranteed Issue rights, which allow him to enroll in Medigap plans A, B, C, F, K, and L. That also means there are certain plans that are not protected by Guaranteed Issue rights. His choices are wider during the Medigap open enrollment period.

Even if he were in perfect health at sixty-seven, the plan that he originally wanted may not even exist at the time that he wants to change into Medigap. Remember that the design of Medigap policies is governed by the Centers for Medicare & Medicaid Services (CMS). That means that CMS also has the right to discontinue plans; it has done this in the past. Plans D, E, H, I, and J no longer exist (although original policy owners still can use their plans as long as they continue to pay premiums).

Medigap and Part B Excess Charges

Earlier, the Medicare Part B Excess charges were explained. Recall that a medical provider can charge up to 15 percent more than the Medicare-allowed charge, and the out-of-pocket costs can be very high. Under Medigap Plan G, the Medicare Part B Excess Charges are covered in full. If you have Plan F or Plan G and the doctor charges more than the Medicare allowed charge, then your Medigap will cover this amount.

For existing policyholders of High-Deductible Plan F, the Part B excess charges are paid after you meet the annual deductible, which is $2,300 in 2019.

We need to examine this particular piece of information because, generally speaking, Plans F and G are more expensive than the other plans. Now, the question is, is the protection provided worth the cost? On one hand, these plans can be approximately $400 more per year in premiums than other Medigap plans. There is no doubt that this is a lot of money.

However, if you are a person with an incurable disease, such as Parkinson's disease, diabetes (type 1), cancer, rheumatoid arthritis, congestive heart failure, or multiple sclerosis, then you are facing a fairly long period in which you will require extensive medical attention.

If you suffer a heart attack requiring open

heart surgery, or if you suffer a stroke, then again, there will be a long, difficult road to recovery. If one episode occurs like this in your lifetime and you incur an Excess Charge, the $400 a year can be recouped many times over, depending on the treatment required.

In addition to the financial considerations, there is also the emotional aspect that has not been mentioned before in this book. People who face serious medical conditions require not only their own strength, but the strength of their support system. Almost no price tag can be put on peace of mind. With Medigap, there will not be an endless trail of medical bills, any worries about how to pay, and any thoughts about the financial costs on those around you. Whether to go with Plan F or G is entirely a consumer's decision.

Foreign Travel

Many of the plans under Medigap actually allow for foreign travel emergency services. There is a $250 deductible. Your Medigap policy will pay for 80 percent of your emergency travel medical expenses, up to a lifetime maximum $50,000. You are responsible for the remainder of the bill. You will probably need to wait to be reimbursed. It may be cumbersome, from a practical point of view, to file a claim while you are in a foreign country, so you will be able to file claims with your insurance company after you return home.

Medigap May Not Be Best

There are situations in which Medicare Advantage may be the better option, when compared to Medigap. As stated in Chapter 6, Medicare Advantage has notably improved in important ways. Intense competition will likely only intensify over time, which means that improvements can be reasonably expected in the future.

As mentioned earlier, Medicare Advantage can offer additional benefits, such as discounts for smoking-cessation programs, weight-loss programs, and vision and dental discounts, among others.[16] While in the short run these may give you some satisfaction, you will quickly forget your discounted trips to the fitness center if you are admitted to the hospital and have large out-of-pocket expenses. You can compare the cost-sharing of Medicare Advantage to Medigap and see for yourself.

You Are Financially Stretched

The phrase "maximize your Medicare" does not mean "minimize your food." Nor does this book suggest that you become insurance poor. You need to eat, pay bills, and live. There are other priorities in life as well. Perhaps you have to support someone else. Maybe you think it is more important to buy clothes for your grandchildren. It isn't the role of *Maximize Your Medicare* to determine this for you. On the other hand, remember that you need to be in good health in order to contribute to others. With that in mind, there are reasons that Medicare Advantage could be a superior choice when compared to Medigap.

You can easily find Medicare Advantage Plans that are cheaper than Medigap. Medicare Advantage is convenient, especially because prescription drug benefits are frequently combined with medical insurance. If you receive prescription drug benefits from another source, like the VA, then the price of a Medicare Advantage Plan without prescription coverage may make sense.

In certain states, HMOs actually rebate you part of your Medicare Part B premium, via your Social Security benefits. While the Part B Excess has been explained, and the risks have also been explained, you may be willing to accept that risk and the inferior cost-sharing arrangements of Medicare Advantage because you need to save the extra money. One objective of this book is to point out that Medigap policies can be found that are essentially the same price as Medicare Advantage Plans, and that due to the consistency of coverage, along with unwritten implications, Medigap is superior to Medicare Advantage. All else equal, then, Medigap would be the better choice.

However, "all else equal" may be language that does not apply to your individual situation. At some price, it may be worth it to accept the inferior cost-sharing terms within Medicare Advantage Plans. Financial priorities may dictate your choices. This is your private financial reality; this book is written so that you know what the implications are of the choices that you make.[17]

You Are Well Over Seventy Years Old

The most popular, most widely available Medigap plans are attained age, which was described earlier in this chapter. Medicare Advantage Plans are entirely community based. That means that premiums of Medicare Advantage do not change, regardless of age. They are reset every year, and it doesn't matter if you are sixty-five or eighty-five — the price is the same.

It may be that the price differential between Medigap and Medicare Advantage, when you reach advanced ages, makes a change from Medigap to Medicare Advantage a very good idea. However, remember that the conditions stated in the section "Base Case: Medigap is Superior to Medicare Advantage" are still true. The language of Medicare Advantage is subject to change, and the premium will change every year. Choosing between Medigap and Medicare Advantage is not easy, and competition has made the decision more challenging. It depends very much on the amount of financial resources you have. If you cannot afford the premiums and find that you are being stretched financially as a result of Medigap premiums as you reach an advanced age, then a change to a Medicare Advantage Plan may be a good idea.

You Always Stay Close to Home

As stated above, one drawback of Medicare Advantage is the idea that there is a network. Cost-sharing is worse (more expensive) if you want to receive services from a provider that is not in your network. In extreme cases (as in an HMO), you would need to bear the entire costs not covered by Original Medicare. In other cases, receiving services from an out-of-network provider can be double (or more) the cost when compared to receiving services from an in-network provider. It is this book's conclusion that the difference between in-network and out-of-network will worsen over time, and in some cases, dramatically.

However, if you do not travel at all, if your providers are the same ones that you have used for a long time, and if the facilities in your area will not change, you may not use the advantages that a Medigap policy offers. In that case, perhaps the extra benefits that often accompany a Medicare Advantage Plan are more worthwhile than the flexibility that you get due to absence of a network. That is up to the consumer.

SWITCHING TO MEDIGAP

State-Specific Medigap Rights

The Medigap open enrollment rules and special enrollment periods apply to every state; there is no dispute about these facts. In addition, some states have provided additional rights to Medicare-eligible residents.

California and Oregon. In certain states,

there is a "Birthday Rule," which allows a current Medigap policyholder to switch carriers to an equivalent or weaker Medigap plan without medical underwriting. As of this writing, California and Oregon are the only two states with this provision.

New York and Connecticut. In these two states, applicants can apply to Medigap at any time during the year. However, you need to be very careful in these locations, because while Medigap enrollment rules are very different, Part D plan eligibility does not change. The safest way to change is to do so during the Annual Election Period, which provides the unrestricted right to enroll in a stand-alone prescription drug plan (Part D), with an effective date of January 1. Then, you can request an effective date of January 1 for Medigap. If executed in this way, you can have both Medigap and Part D begin on the same date, January 1.

Maine. You can switch among Medigap plans at any time during the year.

Missouri. You can switch among Medigap plans within sixty days of the anniversary date of your initial effective date into a Medigap plan.

Minnesota and Wisconsin. Medigap policies in these two states are notably different from other states. In both states, there is a

Basic Plan, and effective add-ons that will pay for other aspects that Original Medicare (Part A and Part B) do not cover.

Washington. In the state of Washington, you can change from any Medigap plan to another, except you cannot change into Medigap Plan A.

Switching from One Medigap Policy to Another

The competition among Medigap carriers is intense. New entrants appear, and existing Medigap carriers may offer additional, non-Medicare benefits that are important to you. For these reasons, you may want to change Medigap carriers.[18]

This is possible, but under most cases, you will be subject to medical underwriting. An insurance company can choose to accept or deny coverage based on your answers to medical questions. See the section "State-Specific Medigap Rights" to see if there are exceptions in your location. That does not mean it is impossible. There can be justifiable reasons for switching Medigap carriers.[19]

It is very important to understand how the application process actually works. Different carriers will have very different decision-making processes. For example, insulin-dependent diabetics or those that have taken certain painkillers may be automatically denied by one carrier, but not by another. The net result is that while you are allowed to apply with many different carriers, that may be unwise. The reason for this is that if you are denied by a specific carrier, then that can become part of your shared record via the MIB, Inc. (see a further description in the Experts' Addendum), and that can result in denials from other insurance companies.

Many people wrongly assume that you can switch Medigap carriers only during the Annual Election Period. That is not true; you can switch from one Medigap carrier to another at any point throughout the year.

SWITCHING FROM MEDICARE ADVANTAGE TO MEDIGAP

Some people do not understand the differences between Medicare Advantage and Medigap and may want to switch after the Medigap open enrollment period has closed. This is possible, but must be done with care, and in this situation, timing and sequence of applying for Medigap is very important.

If you switch during the Annual Election Period (AEP), you will be subject to medical underwriting, unless you qualify for a Special Enrollment Period (SEP). If you do not qualify for Guaranteed Issue, then an insurance company can choose to accept or deny your application, based on your answers to medical questions. If your Medicare Advantage includes prescription drug benefits, then you need to wait for the Annual Election Period, or the open enrollment period, because you will be canceling your prescription drug benefits.

If you cancel your Medicare Advantage Plan during the open enrollment period, which runs from January 1 through February 14, you can cancel your Medicare Advantage Plan and return to Original Medicare, which means that you can select a stand-alone prescription plan (Part D). You will need to be very careful because your application to Medigap may be subject to medical underwriting.

The steps are not difficult, but *it is vital to follow the order* as listed here. Apply for Medigap first and be certain that your application is accepted. Only after your Medigap application has been approved can you enroll in a Part D plan during either the Annual Election Period, which runs from October 15 through December 7, or cancel your Medicare Advantage Plan and enroll in a Part D plan during the open enrollment period, which runs from January 1 through March 31.

SPECIAL TOPICS

It may seem that enrolling in Medigap is easy, and the selection of carriers is irrelevant. However, this chapter has revealed that this may not be the case. This is a short list of other issues that affect Medigap.

Not All Medigap Carriers Are Equal

While Medigap policies are identical to each other, the carriers differ notably. Here are issues to consider.

If you are subject to medical underwriting, then you need to be very careful. The reason is that carriers ask different medical underwriting questions, and underwriting decisions will vary from carrier to carrier. The ripple effect is that if you are rejected by a specific carrier, then it will be more difficult to be accepted by the next carrier. Applications generally ask, "Have you applied for Medigap in the past, and were you rejected?" Only an expert will be able to reasonably guide you in this instance, because an expert should know which carriers will be more likely to accept your application from the beginning.[20]

If you are in excellent health, then you may be better off by selecting a carrier with the most difficult underwriting standards. Why? It has to do with the way that rate increases occur in the future. Future premiums are more likely to rise at a faster rate if you purchase a Medigap policy from a company that does not place restrictions on enrollment. Insurance companies can raise prices based on the claims history of the other policy owners that have the same policy.[21] Therefore, there is no reason to enroll in a policy and be in the same pool with others that are more likely to have a greater incidence of claims, because those higher claims will justify higher premiums in the future. While we have no crystal ball, an expert will have special insight on the underwriting process that occurs at the different carriers in your location.

Plans C and F Are Closing to New Applicants

Medigap is certainly popular, and Plan F has historically been the most dominant plan. However, Plan F and Plan C will no longer be offered to new applicants, beginning on January 1, 2020.[22] In 2013, the first edition of this book strongly suggested that this would be possible, because those two plans paid for the Part B Deductible, which encouraged excessive use of health-care resources. That leaves the government responsible for the 80 percent covered by Medicare Part B, immediately. Both patients and health-care providers would be less likely to seek unnecessary services if the Part B deductible were not paid.

If you are a current policyholder of either Plan C or Plan F, you cannot be involuntarily ejected from your policy. This is one of the features of Medigap: it is *guaranteed renewable,* as long as you continue to pay premiums. The only one that can cancel your Medigap policy is you, and you alone.[23] Note that if you are already enrolled in Medicare Part A and Part B, then you can still apply for Medigap Plan C and F after January 1, 2020. Medigap Plans C and F are closed to those who are not enrolled in both Medicare Part A and Part B prior to January 1, 2020.

Will premiums on Plan F skyrocket because there is an absence of new applicants? There is no easy answer. While this may seem like it makes sense, what must be considered is that the pools of policyholders are being adjusted now. A carrier can reset its pool periodically, without explicitly informing the existing policyholders. Therefore, the idea would be that nothing will really change in the future.

Further, the question is really about the handling of the Part B deductible. Plan F pays for the Part B deductible; Plan G does not. That means that you are responsible for the Part B premium. A little-known fact, however, is that there can be errors in accounting for the Part B premium. Periodically, you will receive a Medicare Summary Notice (MSN) that details the services you received. It will also report to you whether you have satisfied the Part B deductible. The difficulty here is that the accounting function is actually outsourced to a third party, and there can be delays or administrative error. It is my professional experience that errors have been encountered with greater frequency.

The result of these errors is that you can be billed for services that should have been covered by the Medigap carrier. The Medigap carrier only begins paying after the Part B deductible has been satisfied. However, if the accounting does not state that you have satisfied the Part B deductible, then the carrier would not know that it is responsible for any payment. You are then caught in an unenviable crossfire among Medicare, the Medigap carrier, and your health-care provider. This is a definite, unintended consequence, and there is no easy resolution. It is a certainty that this will be an ongoing issue for many, as Plans C and F become unavailable to new applicants.

Preexisting Condition Waiting Period

This quote is from "Choosing a Medigap Policy: A Guide to Health Insurance for People with Medicare" from the Centers for Medicare & Medicaid Services (CMS): "Remember, for Medicare covered services, Original Medicare will still cover the condition, even if the Medigap policy won't cover your out-of-pocket costs, but you're responsible for the coinsurance or copayment."

While the insurance company can't make you wait for your coverage to start, it may be able to make you wait for coverage related to a preexisting condition, which is a health problem you have before the date a new insurance policy starts.

In some cases, the Medigap insurance company can refuse to cover your out-of-pocket costs for these preexisting health problems for up to six months. This is called a "preexisting condition waiting period." After six months, the Medigap policy will cover the preexisting condition. Coverage for a preexisting condition can only be excluded in a Medigap policy if the condition were treated or diagnosed within six months before the date the coverage starts under the Medigap policy. This is called the "look-back period."[24]

If you have no health insurance prior to turning sixty-five, then it may be best to eliminate companies that have the Medigap preexisting condition waiting period. It makes no sense to become Medicare eligible knowing that you require some treatment, waiting for Medicare coverage, just to have coverage by your Medigap plan denied during this waiting period. If your medical situation deteriorates during the first six months after enrolling in Medicare and you require extensive medical attention immediately, then the amount not covered by Medicare Part A and Part B can be large. You will be liable for the cost-sharing under Original Medicare. Remember that if you have had health insurance coverage for the six months prior to Medicare eligibility, this stipulation does not apply to you.

The Bottom Lines

Medigap is the cleanest financial contract you can find. There is no question about the coverage, no language to be misunderstood. There is no network, and the only one that can cancel your Medigap policy is you. It is a question of whether the additional premium, which will be higher than Medicare Advantage in most cases, is worth it. There can be other considerations, such as the additional benefits (health club memberships, dental care, vision care, etc.) and potentially superior prescription drug benefits available via Medicare Advantage.

While it may seem easy and convenient to simply compare premiums today, and randomly apply to Medigap, there are many additional factors to consider, which may affect you in the future. For some people, these factors do not matter. However, those that understand the subtle points in this chapter will know that the difference among carriers may not appear immediately, but in the future. Premiums among carriers do change, especially for those seventy and older, and the difference in premiums can be more than $1,000 a year for the same Medigap plan.

Note: The Medigap policy covers coinsurance only after you have paid the deductible (unless the Medigap policy also covers the deductible).

How to read the chart: If an "X" appears in a column of this chart, the Medi-

TABLE 4. Medigap Plans

	A	B	C	D	F*	G*	K	L	M	N
Medicare part A Coinsurance and hospital costs up to an additional 365 days	x	x	x	x	x	x	x	x	x	x
Medicare Part B Coinsurance or Copayment	x	x	x	x	x	x	50%	75%	x	x
Blood (first 3 pints)	x	x	x	x	x	x	50%	75%	x	x
Part A hospice care coinsurance or copayment	x	x	x	x	x	x	50%	75%	x	x
Skilled Nursing Facility (SNF) care coinsurance			x	x	x	x	50%	75%	x	x
Medicare Part A deductible		x	x	x	x	x	50%	75%	50%	x
Medicare Part B deductible			x		x		50%	75%		
Medicare Part B Excess Charges					x	x				
Foreign travel emergency (up to plan limits)			80%	80%	80%	80%			80%	80%
Out of pocket limit							$5,560	$2,780		

gap policy covers 100 percent of the described benefit. If a row lists a percentage, the policy covers that percentage of the described benefit. If a row is blank, the policy doesn't cover that benefit.

Plan F and Plan G have high-deductible options (F*) and (G*). If you choose these options, you are responsible for the entire high-deductible amount before your Medigap plan pays anything. This amount is determined annually by the CMS. Once satisfied, high-deductible Plans F and G will cover all costs after Original Medicare, including Part B Excess charges, if applicable.

Plan N pays 100 percent of the Part B coinsurance, except for a copayment of up to a maximum of $20 for some office visits and up to a maximum of $50 copayment for emergency-room visits.

Plan K and Plan L have an out-of-pocket limit of $5,560 and $2,780, respectively, in 2019. These levels adjust annually.

Chapter 7
Working Beyond Sixty-Five

People Are Working Longer

This is no surprise to anyone, because Social Security Full Retirement Age (FRA) is now sixty-six and is gradually increasing to sixty-seven. The inevitable result is that people will continue to work beyond sixty-five. The ripple effects are enormous because it greatly complicates the transition to Medicare. The simple reason is that although people may work beyond sixty-five, Medicare eligibility remains unchanged. A much more complicated combination of choices regarding Medicare has emerged, and there is no going back.

An aging, working population means that employers and employees will face challenges, choices, and combinations that have not been well understood, well documented, or carefully considered. The anecdotal evidence is overwhelming. For employers large and small, the choices being made affect the financial well-being of the company, active employees, and retirees. Unfortunately, the widespread mishandling of these new combinations has left employers with financial costs that could have been avoided and has left employees with inferior coverage and excessively expensive premiums.

Errors being made make this the single most important segment of this book. Benefits at the workplace have weakened notably.[1] When combined with the federal regulations that are in favor of the Medicare eligible, and the benefits described in Chapters 3 through 6, a full understanding of this chapter can result in much better coverage, at the right cost. Not examining these combinations? Costly to employees, employers, and the economy as a whole.

Can Employees Delay Enrollment in Medicare?

If you are working and covered by health insurance provided by your employer, then you can delay enrollment in Medicare Part A, Medicare Part B, and Medicare Part D.[2] It is usually the case that people enroll in Part A since it has no premium. If a person has an HSA bank account, special care must be taken here, because you cannot contribute to an HSA and simultaneously receive

Part A benefits (you can withdraw for health-related expenses at any age).[3]

If your health insurance includes prescription drug benefits, then you can delay enrollment in Medicare Part D for sixty-three days. Sixty-three days is the maximum number of days that you can be without prescription drug benefits and avoid the Part D Late Enrollment Penalty, if you are sixty-five years old or older or enrolled in Medicare Part A. It is very important to understand that prescription coverage received must be independently certified by the CMS as "creditable coverage." It is also very important to understand that while you can delay, that it doesn't mean you should. Chapter 8 addresses this complicated topic.

Employer-Sponsored Enrollment Calendar

Special care is required regarding the election periods when an employer-sponsored group plan is involved. The reason is that employer-sponsored group plans frequently have enrollment periods that are different from Medicare. For example, many large employer-sponsored group plans have enrollment periods that end after Medicare's Annual Election Period (AEP, October 15 through December 7). You can disregard this period if you are covered by employer-sponsored health insurance because you will have a Special Enrollment Period (SEP) when you can elect a Medicare Advantage Plan or a Part D plan.[4] If you are not enrolled in Medicare Part B, then your Medigap application will be approved under Medigap open enrollment rules.

This can be very confusing. Canceling employer-sponsored health insurance can be done, but special care needs to be taken because there are enrollment deadlines in effect if you want to enroll in Medicare Part B (eight months), Medicare Part D (sixty-three days), Medicare Advantage (the date that Part B is effective), and Medigap (six months after Medicare Part B is effective). This is a very convoluted combination. The best approach is simple. Simply avoid all of these different dates by making certain that the effective date of Medicare Part B, Medicare Advantage, or Part D and Medigap is the day after employer-sponsored coverage ends.

Procrastinators make the error of waiting until the last moment before deciding upon the right configuration of benefits (group vs. Medicare, etc.). If you wait too long, the selection can be made for you, and you will be left with Original Medicare. Be careful.

SMALL EMPLOYER

For employees at small employers, choosing to remain enrolled in a small-group plan is odd, because the premium is very likely to be far costlier, and the coverage is very likely weaker. A further explanation of this will be provided later in this chapter. There are going to be exceptions that need to be examined, related to other benefits or family members that require coverage under the employee's group coverage. There can be exceptions due to innovations that are occurring in the insurance market.[5]

Employees can enroll, without premium, in Medicare Part A, as long as they are eligible. Employees may choose to enroll in Medicare Part B, or they can choose to delay.

If the employee at a small-group employer (defined as fewer than twenty full-time employees) enrolls in either Part A or Part B, then Medicare is primary, and the group-sponsored health insurance plan will be secondary. Special care will need to be taken here, because the prescription drug benefits must be certified to be "creditable," which means that it is as least as good as Medicare Part D, and that certification comes from the CMS. There will be an explicit explanation in a "Summary of Benefits."

Base Case: Medicare Is Superior

It is unlikely that delaying a private Medicare configuration is a good idea. This fits neither the single employee nor the employer. The combined premiums of Medicare Part A, Part B, and Part D (with Medicare Advantage and/or Medigap) are very likely to be thousands of dollars a year lower than the overall cost of small employer group health insurance. Therefore, there would need to be a circumstance that exists if you decide to stay enrolled in small employer group-sponsored health insurance.[6]

This Happens: Single, Active Employee at Small Company

A small employer offers health insurance to full-time employees and pays 50 percent of the total premium. For the newly turned sixty-five-year-old employee, that premium is approximately $900, of which the employer pays $450, and the employee would be responsible for $450.

Why? The employee could pay $135.50 for Part B and elect either a Medicare Advantage or Medigap Plan (and Part D, if Medigap were elected). The premium, deductibles, copays, and coinsurance under Medicare would all be vastly superior to small-group health insurance at that premium level. Medicare Advantage costs between $0 and $100 a month. Medigap would cost approximately $140 (average across the nation) and $33 for Part D.

Instead, the employer is not properly informed, and the employee does not know that these are the comparable premiums. The coverage of Medicare Advantage or Medicare will likely be dramatically superior to the small group health insurance plan. The small-group plan would definitely not be a Platinum plan under the ACA; it would be a Gold plan, at best.

Exceptions for Employees at Small Employers[7]

There can be exceptions to this base case. The simple reason is that the active employee at a small employer may be enrolled in an employer-sponsored group health insurance plan in order to cover other family members. Let's take a look.

First, let us assume that a spouse is Medicare eligible. Then, the base case will almost certainly apply. In fact, if the employee cancels his or her group-sponsored coverage, then the spouse will gain access to a Special Enrollment Period, including Guaranteed Acceptance into Medigap plans

A, K, and L.

If the spouse is not eligible for Medicare, there are multiple options:

Spouse can enroll in an individual health insurance plan. The spouse will be issued it automatically, since the spouse's coverage will have ended because the employee has canceled. Depending on the household income and the state of residence, the spouse could also obtain a subsidy under Medicaid expansion rules.

Spouse can choose to not enroll in health insurance or purchase a short-term medical plan if the spouse is turning sixty-five in the near future.

Why would a spouse choose to not enroll? Money. At small employers, the cost of covering the spouse can be very expensive. In some cases, not enrolling is necessary because the spouse has medical issues and does not qualify for Medicaid expansion, and the cost of individual health insurance makes it impractical. So there is no other choice. That does not mean that it does not deserve examination of the issues, and the math of money.

LARGE EMPLOYER

Employees can enroll, without premium, in Medicare Part A. Employees may choose to enroll in Medicare Part B, or they can choose to delay. Employees at large employers usually choose to delay, since at large employers, the group-sponsored plan is primary, and Medicare is secondary. For many, the cost of Part B is not worth the secondary coverage.

Private, individual investigation here can provide tremendous value to both the employee and employers. There is no shortcut to examining the details. Do not rely on others to confirm this information. Confirm it yourself by locating the language in the "Summary of Benefits" of the employer-sponsored plan. Sometimes, human resource departments do not spell this out for you clearly. When you contact your human resources or employee benefit department, ask the human resources person to point out the location where the language exists in the "Summary of Benefits" that explains the requirement to enroll in Medicare Part B. While you can blame the human resources department for its human error, the one paying the higher cost will be . . . you. It is highly unlikely that you will have any recourse to your (former) employer if the HR department informs you incorrectly. The quality of the answers that you receive can vary wildly, which is why obtaining written evidence is important.

Base Case: Employees at Large Employers Should Delay

For many, the employer-sponsored group plan, for active employees, is the best plan. The overriding reason may be the premium. At large employers, employees are not required to pay the Medicare Part B premium, since the large group coverage is primary. (For Medicare purposes, a "large employer" is one that exceeds twenty full-time employees. Notably, the definition of "large employer" is different under Affordable Care Act rules.)

In addition, large-group plans might contain a prescription drug benefits coverage gap, as described in Chapter 4. If there is no coverage gap, then the employer-sponsored plan may be the best option. Your total cost of protection may be lower under an employer-sponsored group plan, even if that means that there are unfavorable co-payments and deductibles for health services you receive from a physician or hospital.

It will entirely depend on the specific details in the large-group plan. Large-group insurance will be subject to change. The issue this raises is that your total cost can increase, meaning your copayment and deductible schedules can all increase, and you will have no control over it. This will be governed by the agreement between the employer and the insurance company.

Notably, it is likely that large employers could establish provisions to help both employer and employee, by simply creating acceptable incentives for the employee to cancel his or her large-employer group-sponsored coverage, enroll in Medicare Part B, and adopt a privately purchased Medicare configuration.

For example, certain large employers provide a financial payment to those that do not elect to participate in employer-sponsored coverage. Given the changing demographic of the workforce, creative ideas will be required in order to deal with the rising cost of health insurance and the financial value provided via Medicare.

Exceptions for Employees at Large Employers[8]

There are certainly exceptions to the base case for active employees for large employers. Let's take a look at a few examples.

Premium Charged for Spouse Is Too High

This should be self-evident. At certain large employers, the premium charged for spousal coverage does not make sense, when comparing the monthly premium of the spousal coverage to Medicare. It is very unlikely that the actual coverage under a group plan is superior to that of Medigap. (In fact, this is almost impossible.)

High Deductibles/Out-of-Pocket Maximum

This is a pure math-of-money exercise. While the premiums would look to be lower under a large-group employer-sponsored plan, the language of group plans is almost certainly weaker than both Medicare Advantage and Medigap/Part D. For example, large-group plans have deductibles and out-of-pocket maximums that are usually much, much higher than those under Medicare Advantage. You already have read that in most cases, the cost of medical services under Medicare is limited to the Part B deductible, $198 in 2020.

It is very important to note that when a married couple/family has coverage under the employee, then there is likely to be a combined "household deductible," or "household out-of-pocket maximum," and that the total out-of-pocket expenses for the household are high but never hit the out-of-pocket maximum. In this instance, the total costs of large group employer-sponsored health insurance can be much higher than Medicare.

While the premium may look lower, if it is a certainty that you face ongoing health-care services, then the total cost to you may be higher by staying with the large-group employer-sponsored plan. That is especially the case if the employer pays you for canceling your participation in the group plan.

Spouse in Exceptional Health

If the spouse is eligible for Medicare, then the spouse should independently decide whether Medicare or coverage as the spouse is superior. One should not assume anything: this book reveals that Medicare Advantage and Medigap/Part D are likely to be vastly superior to the coverage of any other health insurance.

If the spouse is not eligible for Medicare, there are multiple options:

Spouse can enroll in an individual health insurance plan. The spouse will be issued it automatically, since the spouse's coverage will have ended because the employee has canceled. Depending on the household income and the state of residence, the spouse could also obtain a subsidy under Medicaid expansion rules.

Spouse can choose not to enroll in health

insurance or purchase a short-term medical plan if the spouse is turning sixty-five in the near future.

Spouse with High Health-Care Requirements

This is a very, very special situation. Since the spouse cannot belong to the large-group plan without the employee, dropping that plan will result in a loss of coverage for the spouse. Carriers will not allow a spouse of an employee (or retiree) to remain covered if the employee is not. If the spouse is not Medicare-eligible, this would be a Qualifying Life Event as defined by the ACA. The spouse can enroll in an ACA-compliant plan and, depending on household income, receive a subsidy to assist payments of premiums, copays/coinsurance, or both.[9]

For Medicare-eligible spouses, this is effectively cancellation of the spouse's coverage, which creates an SEP for the spouse. Since the spouse is entitled to a Special Enrollment Period, the spouse can enroll in any Medicare Advantage or Medigap plan without medical underwriting, and a standalone Part D plan. This is not a misprint. A spouse could have a preexisting condition and be accepted for Medigap under Medigap Guaranteed Issue rules in this instance.

Employer Group Plans and the Coverage Gap ("Donut Hole")

The important question about the donut hole is how it may be better or worse than your existing prescription plan. In certain large employer-sponsored plans, there is no concept of donut hole. If your drug costs are very high, the prescription drug costs may be cheaper under your employer-provided group plan, when compared to a stand-alone Part D (prescription drug plan), or MAPD plan.

As a result, you may want to stay with your employer plan. However, it isn't always that simple. Sometimes people say, "I want to stay with my employer due to the fact that the drug cost will be lower." This may be true, or not. Do not assume that the best case is staying with your employer-provided plan. If you conclude that this is the case, after asking the right questions, then it is fine for you to stay with it.

Even if there is no donut hole, it may not be entirely clear that this is reason enough to stay with an employer-sponsored group plan. Your prescription savings need to be compared to the savings that you might have gotten on superior medical plans in the private market. Remember, medical coverage in the private market is frequently superior to the coverage in a group plan. Therefore, your employer-provided medical benefits must be weighed against the medical plan that you would have under a Medicare Advantage or a Medigap plan. On balance, the medical coverage and cost-sharing arrangement under a Medicare Advantage Prescription Drug (MAPD) plan or Medigap plan may be worth the extra cost. That must be done on a case-by-case basis, and there is no shortcut to it.

An advisor or an agent may be useful in this case because he/she would be able to add up the plans' costs, as well as their benefits, for you so that you choose the best overall plan. It is vital that Medicare-eligible persons understand that the two components (medical and prescription) be considered in combination, and not one without regard to the other.

The reason it is important to consider both the prescription plan and medical plan together is that if you are concerned about the high cost of prescriptions, it is usually the case that you have a medical situation that requires constant attention. For others, this is not the case; the cost of prescriptions may be the entirety.

One common mistake is that people ignore the correlation between prescription costs and the medical services they require. The reason that people get rejected by private insurance companies before becoming Medicare eligible is that insurance companies do not make this mistake. Insurance companies know, given a list of medications, that further medical services will be required in the future if a person takes multiple medications.

If You Decide to Cancel

If you choose to cancel employer-sponsored coverage, you must have the person or department at your employer who is responsible for benefits administration complete an official form, CMS-L564E.[10] When your employer-sponsored group coverage ends, you will have eight months to enroll in Medicare Part B. If you delay enrollment beyond the eight-month deadline, you will face a Medicare Part B Late Enrollment Penalty originally described in Chapter 3.

It is important to note that this is entirely different from the time that you are required to have prescription drug benefits that are deemed to be creditable coverage by the CMS. For prescription drug benefits, the longest period that you can be without prescription drug benefits, and enrolled in Medicare Part A, is sixty-three days. This can be very confusing for those that procrastinate.

The Bottom Line

These are the complicated situations that an increasing number of Americans will face. The number of possible results is enormous. The pressure on all parties (employers, employees, retirees, spouses) is largely unavoidable, as people retire later and work longer.

While "used to work," and "that's the way it has always been," are convenient phrases, they are now obsolete. Expert guidance can help you avoid overlooking a critical factor in decision-making.

The bottom line is that if a Medicare-eligible person and/or the spouse have access to employer-provided health insurance, there is no shortcut to doing the math. This conclusion is dominating our professional experience.

CHAPTER 8
RETIREE BENEFIT PLANS

TRUTHS AND MYTHS

Myth: You cannot change from an employer-sponsored retiree plan to a privately purchased Medicare Advantage or Medigap plan.

Truth: Employer-sponsored retiree plans are weakening as a result of demographic and financial pressure facing employers, both large and small.

Truth: You need to be very careful if canceling, because rejoining a retiree plan is not guaranteed by the employer. There is no regulation to protect you. If you wanted to rejoin a retiree plan, it is at the discretion of the employer.

For a variety of reasons, retiree health benefits are being reduced at a rapid rate, and this can be very unsettling to retirees. This weakening has taken two forms. First, employers are choosing to weaken retiree plans via higher premiums or weaker benefits. Second, some employers have ceased to offer retiree benefits altogether.[1] For retirees, the issue is that they may have wrongly assumed that retiree health benefits were a guaranteed part of an overall retirement benefits package.[2]

Corporations and government entities (city, county, state) are struggling mightily under the financial weight of their Other Post-Retirement Employee Benefits (OPEB) obligations.[3] The number of retirees at many employers is greater than the number of active employees. Despite the discomfort, this reality won't change anytime soon.

Now, the surprise — this may be better for you, the consumer. What is important to remember is that if your retiree health benefits are canceled, you will be granted a Special Enrollment Period (SEP), which may actually improve the range of options that you can select in the private market. Chapters 4 through 7 immediately apply to you.

The second surprise? Retiree health benefits may actually be weaker than Medicare Advantage or Medigap and Part D today, even if your retiree health benefits are unchanged. The simple reason for this? Insurance company competition has become extremely competitive, and the result is that the benefits and premiums can compare very favorably against your retiree health benefits.

The most important takeaways of this chapter are the following:

- Do not panic if your retiree health benefits are canceled.
- Compare your existing retiree health benefits versus Medicare Advantage, Medigap, and Part D available in your geographic location. Do not assume that your existing retiree benefits are superior to those available to the public.

RETIREMENT FROM A SMALL EMPLOYER

For Medicare purposes, a small employer is defined as a company with fewer than twenty full-time employees.[4] COBRA is not available at small employers, which requires at least twenty full-time employees. If COBRA coverage is not available, you can have sixty-three days with prescription drug coverage without the Part D Late Enrollment Penalty. This is very confusing for consumers, because you can have no health insurance coverage for eight months without the penalty, but you can have no prescription coverage for only sixty-three days.

At small employers, retiree health benefits are almost nonexistent. While they are made available by carriers, the reasoning for sponsoring a small employer retiree health benefits segment does not usually make sense, for the employer or the retiree. A largely unknown fact is that group retiree policies exist for small employers, which have benefits equivalent or superior to privately available Medicare Advantage. In addition, there are group retiree policies that mimic Medigap coverage and can be combined with prescription drug benefits superior to the stand-alone prescription plans described in Chapter 4.[5]

RETIREMENT FROM A LARGE EMPLOYER

For Medicare purposes, a large employer is defined as a company with more than twenty full-time employees. If you retire, you have eight months to enroll in Part B, from the date your coverage ends, without penalty. That doesn't mean that you should delay; it only means that you can. This has been described in Chapter 1, "Enrollment."

If you are married to a spouse that is not Medicare eligible and you cannot identify health insurance that matches the premium and coverage under COBRA, this can be reason to retain COBRA coverage for eight months. In the overwhelming number of cases, COBRA coverage usually includes prescription drug benefits that qualify as creditable coverage, and therefore you can avoid the Part D Late Enrollment Penalty during this time. However, once that eight months expires, COBRA cannot be the reason for delaying enrollment in Part B. Delaying enrollment in Part B will subject you to the Part B Late Enrollment Penalty.

The Base Case

For retirees of large employers, an employer-sponsored retiree plan may be the best plan. The overriding reason may be the price. At certain large employers, retirees may not be required to pay the Medicare Part B premium, since the large group coverage is primary.[6] However, if the group retiree benefits plan is a group Medicare Advantage Plan, then enrollment in Medicare Part A and Medicare Part B will be required.

Large group plans might contain a prescription drug benefits coverage gap, as described in Chapter 4. If there is no coverage gap, the employer-sponsored plan may be the best option. Your total cost of coverage may be lower under an employer-sponsored group plan, even if that means that there are unfavorable copayments and deductibles for health services you receive from a physician or hospital. It will entirely depend on the math of money comparison. A complete examination of the options available should take place with someone fully up to date on Medigap plans, who is also able to thoroughly analyze the employer-sponsored plans.

These are the key takeaways:

- Large employer retiree health benefits need to be very clearly superior to the private Medicare options, because there is the risk that the retiree plans will weaken, for reasons beyond the retiree's control. That will leave the retiree with limited options, at precisely the wrong time.
- Coverage for family members (spouse, children) may be a very good reason for keeping an otherwise-inferior retiree health benefits plan.
- It is vital to understand your employer's working policy to see if you can change your mind and revert to your employer-sponsored retiree health plan.[7] While it is very unlikely that

retiree benefits improve due to pressures mentioned here, you may have a specific reason to switch back.

These takeaways are frequently ignored or violated. Let's take some real-life examples.

This Happens: A Bankrupt Company

Company D is under the auspices of the Pension Benefit Guaranty Corporation (PBGC). It offers a group plan for retirees that is similar to that of Medigap as well as a prescription drug plan, and this company requires enrollment in Medicare Part B. The prescription drug plan has the same provisions as Medicare Part D, which means that it also includes a coverage gap. The employer also charges a monthly premium that includes both the drug and medical plans.

The problem here is that the total cost of the additional amounts charged on a monthly basis, on top of the Part B deductible, begins at $160 a month. In this particular case, the medical coverage is no better than what exists in the Medigap market. It is more expensive and provides fewer benefits. Nevertheless, retirees stay with this disadvantageous plan.

This Happens: A Global, Thriving Company

Sometimes, the reason an employer-sponsored retiree benefit plan may seem cheaper is that the employer has put in money from its own funds in order to keep the prices low, to the benefit of its retirees. However, the employer may not be under the obligation to do so, and it can discontinue this type of subsidy if the funds reserved for this purpose have been depleted. To make matters worse, legacy collective bargaining agreements, due to mergers and acquisitions, have restricted companies from renegotiating costly retiree health benefit plans.

If this is the case, premiums may increase substantially. Your "Summary of Benefits" may well describe a situation where the company can choose to discontinue the subsidy and increases are passed to the retiree. The net effect of this type of employer-sponsored retiree group plan is that the benefits and costs are no better than what exists in the private market, and the costs may in certain cases be more expensive.

This situation is real, and many persons who have been dedicated employees to a particular employer for a long period may be disappointed. But given the pressures on treasury departments of large corporations, the scenario can easily be the case.

Medicare Retiree and Non-Medicare Spouse

There are certain situations where you will need to stay with your employer-sponsored retiree group plan, even if it is more expensive, and even if your cost-sharing terms are worse than what is available under a Medicare Advantage or Medigap plan. The primary situation is when the retiree is married to a non-Medicare eligible person. The large majority of group plans do not allow a retiree to disenroll and keep the spouse on the employer-sponsored plan.

If that is the case, then the question is whether the spouse is eligible for private health insurance. Under the ACA, the spouse is always eligible to enroll in private health insurance under a Qualifying Life Event (QLE) and, potentially, financial assistance toward health insurance premiums, depending on location. So the question will be whether this makes financial sense.

There is no longer the requirement for an individual to be enrolled in health insurance. There is no tax penalty if you do not have health insurance. In a way, this adds an additional, potentially simpler path for married couples. A Medicare-eligible person can retire, and the spouse can choose to not purchase health insurance or buy a noncompliant plan (like a short-term medical/cancer/stroke/heart attack indemnity plan). That is the choice of the household and not necessarily the recommendation of this book.

The reason this deserves mention is the spouse may be able to obtain health insurance at a cheaper rate than the price being charged by the employer; the spouse is charged more than the employee in group plans. It works this way to prevent people from staying in their jobs or retiree plan simply to obtain health insurance for the spouse.

Retiree and Medicare-Eligible Spouse

You cannot delay enrollment in Medicare if you are the spouse of a retiree. It does not matter if the retiree is Medicare eligible or not. A Medicare-eligible spouse can only delay enrollment in Medicare Part B if the spouse is married to an active employee and is added under the employee's health insurance. Admittedly, this is complicated, but this point must be understood in order to avoid late enrollment penalties.

When does this apply? If the employee is not yet Medicare eligible, then retires, and is covered by retiree health benefits, this immediately becomes important. The spouse, if he/she is over the age of sixty-five, must enroll in Medicare Part A, Part B, and Part D (or be covered by creditable prescription drug coverage).

If Your Employer Cancels Retiree Health Benefits

It can be the case that an employer simply stops providing retiree health benefits. This has happened, this is happening (and being actively considered), and it will happen. There can be little or no advance warning. You probably know someone that has received this type of notification in the mail.

First, do not panic. You will be allowed to select a Medicare Advantage or a Medigap plan, along with a Medicare Part D plan, if necessary, under a Special Enrollment Period (SEP). From the date of discontinuation, you will have sixty-three days to select a new prescription drug plan. You will have eight months to enroll in Part B without incurring a penalty.

You need to be careful here because the rules are different if you want to select a

Medicare Advantage Plan that includes prescription drug benefits, because you only have sixty-three days from the time that a retiree health plan is canceled until you must enroll in a prescription drug plan that is deemed to be creditable coverage.

These dates are very confusing, which can be highly distressing. Best way to manage these moving dates? Don't delay, so that you can avoid the confusion of when late enrollment penalties and Special Enrollment Periods apply, and when those dates pass.

Second, you will need to keep the copy of the notice of cancellation from your employer and/or the insurance company that provided the employer-sponsored health benefits. In your "Summary of Benefits," or in a separate document, there will be a Letter of Creditable Coverage. This will be necessary to use as evidence of your eligibility for a Special Enrollment Period. In order to enroll in any plan — Medicare Advantage, Medigap, or Part D — this document will need to be forwarded to the insurance carrier you choose.

This Happens

A globally recognized company has declared bankruptcy during the early 2000s. Salaried employees, not protected from bankruptcy, have employee benefits slowly, but inevitably, taken from them. Finally, retiree health benefits are next. Medicare-eligible, white-collar workers are given a stipend as a substitute for health benefits, and they attend coordinated employee information sessions. Many employees accept the recommendations and enroll in the Medigap policy presented during these sessions. Now, that insurance company faces severe claims over time, and rates have gone up multiple times a year. Those with preexisting conditions are largely ineligible from switching to other carriers (insurance companies), because the open enrollment period is over, and the Special Enrollment Period has also expired. The retiree now can choose to either accept rapidly rising premiums or a plan with weaker coverage.

EMPLOYER-SPONSORED MEDICARE ADVANTAGE

When you become Medicare eligible, it is vital to know what plan the employer is providing to you. It can be the case that the employer is enrolling you in a Medicare Advantage Plan whose network may not be the same as the plan you were using prior to Medicare eligibility. It will certainly be the case that you will be required to enroll in Medicare Part B: this is always the case if you want to enroll in any Medicare Advantage Plan, in any market.

The confusing part of this is that the Medicare plan that you were given as a retiree can be different from the HMO or PPO that you were given as an active employee in your pre-Medicare days. That means that the list of providers might not be the same that covered you before you were Medicare eligible.[8]

This is a very important point, and as a result you need to consider carefully what you are actually doing, and what you were actually electing. If you travel out of the state frequently, or for many months during the year, you can end up finding out that your total medical costs, meaning your premiums plus out-of-pocket expenses, may exceed other arrangements which could be done in the private market, where there may be no such restrictions. That will entirely depend on which plans are made available by your employer.

Dental, Vision, and Other Benefits

Some retirees believe that there are other types of additional benefits as part of the employer-sponsored plan that are very important, such as dental and vision insurance. There is a great deal of confusion about dental and vision insurance. The reality is that dental and vision insurance is often limited by a maximum amount of benefits that can be received in a calendar year. However, the premiums available in the large employer group market are frequently less expensive than the premiums in the private market.[9]

For those people who require extensive dental work, for example, you will find that the annual benefit amounts can be somewhere in the $1,000 to $1,500 range, per year, per person. As a result, the amount of benefit actually received by the retiree and their family members is very limited. That is up to the consumer to decide.

Remember that you need to pay very careful attention to enrollment issues, such as your ability to rejoin a retiree benefits plan later. In many cases, rejoining retiree plans is not allowed. However, there is no written regulation on the matter; it is purely case by case.

What Employers Can Do

This topic is too broad to cover in one section. However, there are some guidelines to follow. First, both employers and employees can be better off if employers create incentives for employees to elect a Medicare plan or Medigap plan independently.[10] This may require negotiation of existing contracts. Nevertheless, the savings could be well worth it.

Second, Health Savings Accounts (HSAs) are a good way to incentivize employees to maintain their health, and to lower costs. They can be established so that if someone needs to defer election of Medicare Part B, that person may be able to save extra money on a pretax basis, which can in turn be used to pay for Medicare Part B premiums when he/she enrolls in Medicare Part B. One of the group health plan alternatives should include a High Deductible Health Plan, which works alongside a Health Savings Account. Note that there are complications for some, because employees cannot contribute to HSAs and be enrolled in Medicare Part A: there will be tax consequences.

CONCLUSIONS

We are not going to settle the debate over statements like "companies owe retirees these benefits," "employers should not neglect their responsibilities to retirees," "we built this company, we worked for decades," etc. This book is dealing with the way things actually are, and the way that things are very likely to work in the future.

If employer and employees work together, the difference in pricing between group retiree health plans and Medicare plans (either group Medicare Advantage or Medigap/Part D) is so large that the cost savings are worth the effort. For small employers, this pressure usually does not exist. For large employers, this is notably different. There are many instances, however, when the rational solution remains elusive. Employer/employee relations become strained, reasonableness is discarded, and both sides suffer. These days, this can be easily found in the case of municipalities, where fiscal concerns are clashing with legacy collective bargaining agreements. Mergers and acquisitions are also creating pressure.

Unionized employees and their employer, a local government under financial duress, are renegotiating their collective bargaining agreement. Some agreements stipulate that retirees are entitled to identical coverage that they received when they were active employees. Now, Medicare Advantage and Medigap are superior in both price and coverage to the benefits these retirees were receiving when they were active employees. However, the union and management cannot find a middle ground, and the active employees go on strike.

For employers, retiree health-benefit expenses can threaten the viability of the company or reduce services that a municipality/state provides to the general public. For retirees, the message is that the private market may provide both superior benefits at similar premiums. This is the result of the intense competition that exists among carriers. It is very frequently overlooked by retirees at large companies. Not only are the prices lower, but the coverage is often superior to that offered by a group retiree benefits health.

Perhaps both sides can all agree on one thing: an employer choosing to close due to the high cost of health insurance for those over sixty-five is the least favorable outcome. Yet, those are the stakes. As such, everything should be explored fully. If you are an employer, and you have Medicare-eligible employees or retirees, then you should attempt to find a better solution. It is very likely that you will.

CHAPTER 9
SPECIAL GROUPS

TRUTHS AND MYTHS

Myth: Retiree groups always provide benefits that are superior to Medigap and privately purchased Medicare Advantage Plans.

Truth: The Veterans Administration recommends that veterans enroll in Medicare Part B when turning sixty-five years old.

There are many large groups of Medicare beneficiaries. If you are part of one of these groups, then there are additional factors to consider.

VETERANS ADMINISTRATION (VA)

VA benefits, including retiree health benefits, are a very complicated matter. There are advantages, as well as drawbacks, to the VA medical system for those who are eligible for Medicare.

The Department of Veterans Affairs recommends that veterans enroll in Medicare Part A and Part B. Among the reasons for this is that the level of funding of VA benefits is not guaranteed in the future. The most recent episodes of long waiting lists for veterans to receive health care can be added to those reasons.

Eligibility and cost-sharing are subject to review by the VA. If you have been receiving VA benefits in the past, that may not necessarily be the case in the future. There have been cases when a person previously receiving limited benefits from the VA has been stripped of these benefits, which left the Medicare-eligible beneficiary in a position in which he had to find both health insurance and prescription insurance.

Strictly speaking, veterans that receive medical care at VA medical centers (or those facilities that are contracted to provide VA service) are not required to enroll in Medicare Part B. However, if you fall into that category and attempt to enroll in Part B later, you will be subject to the Part B Late Enrollment Penalty described in Chapter 3.

Further, veterans that receive prescriptions from the VA are not required to enroll in Medicare Part D. As many know, prescription drug benefits through the VA are frequently superior to Medicare Part D, due to the very low copays associated with the VA. That said, some veterans find the process of refilling prescriptions through the VA to be difficult (they are too far away need to see VA primary-care physician). There is no conflict between having both VA prescription drug benefits and a Medicare Part D plan.

For veterans, there are Medicare Advantage Plans that are almost certainly intended for them. In Chapter 5, additional benefits were described as part of certain Medicare Advantage and/or Medicare Advantage Prescription Drug (MAPD) plans. An easy example would be possible discounts for smoking-cessation programs. It is entirely possible for a veteran to enroll in Medicare Part B, use VA benefits for health and prescriptions for maintenance purposes, and have a Medicare Advantage Plan that does not include prescription drug benefits (health only). Medicare Advantage carriers have added many benefits in the form of lower copays and deductibles. That will allow you to access the health club memberships and other perks for Medicare Advantage policyholders.

Additionally, you can use the Medicare Advantage card (although there will be cost-sharing in accordance with the Medicare

Advantage or MAPD plan) if you strongly prefer to not use VA facilities. If you have an "emergency" that is not ruled to qualify as an emergency, then you would have a lower out-of-pocket cost by using your Medicare Advantage Plan.

This Happens

A VA beneficiary goes to the emergency room at a local hospital, which is not a VA hospital, with the belief that he is very ill. It turns out to be nothing. He is required to pay the full cost of the services administered at the emergency room. The only portion that is reimbursed is the ambulance transfer from the non-VA facility to the VA facility, and then only if coordinated by the VA facility.

TRICARE FOR LIFE (TFL)[1]

For career military retirees, the most comprehensive set of benefits is called Tricare for Life (TFL); career military retirees are entitled to a full set of benefits. In addition, it has been the case that those people who suffered a disability that is directly linked to active combat may be granted TFL. The most prevalent case is when someone has a documented case of exposure to Agent Orange and has suffered from a medical situation that has been linked to that exposure. Sometimes, TFL is not granted. The best way to find out if you are entitled to TFL is to contact the Veterans Administration.

Tricare for Life requires enrollment in both Medicare Part A and Part B. TFL beneficiaries may have some small copays for prescriptions and will also have complete medical coverage. That medical coverage is based on the military set of approved procedures and treatments.[2]

If you do qualify for TFL, you can additionally have a Medicare Advantage Plan. Depending on the plan, that can mean that you can take advantage of dental benefits, vision benefits, and other services, such as chiropractic services. There are an increasing number of Medicare Advantage Plans that have vouchers for health-related items, as well as credits toward the Part B premium, as discussed in Chapter 5.

Disabled

If you are entitled to Medicare prior to the age of sixty-five, due to receiving two years of Social Security Disability Insurance benefits, then there are some very important points to remember. The exact timing is explained in Chapter 1, under the heading

"Eligibility Prior to Sixty-Five Years Old." You will not necessarily receive the full information regarding your rights when you become entitled to Medicare in this case. This can lead to a number of problems, which can be reasonably avoided.

First, if Part D initial enrollment period has opened and you do not have prescription drug coverage that is deemed to be creditable coverage by the CMS, then you can be assessed the Part D Late Enrollment Penalty. You will not receive a notice regarding the Part D Late Enrollment Penalty until you attempt to enroll in a Part D or MAPD plan.

Second, eligibility for Medicare Part A and Part B also implies that Medicare Advantage can be elected per the normal Medicare Advantage enrollment rules. That means that the ICEP, Annual Election Period, and the Open Enrollment Period apply. It is very, very likely that a Medicare Advantage Plan will be superior to any individual health insurance contract available from any other source, even if you received a subsidy due to Medicaid expansion rules under the ACA.

Third, Medigap is usually not available for those who are eligible for Medicare prior to the age of sixty-five. There is no federal rule that provides this right. However, there can be certain states that require carriers to offer Medigap plans to those younger than sixty-five. You will need to check your state. Many financial representatives are unaware of the exceptions.

Fourth, when a disabled person turns sixty-five, he or she is entitled to something that carriers call "ICEP2." It translates to "second bite of the apple." That means a disabled person can enroll in Medigap and Part D, at the best possible rates available in the location of residence. There would be no medical underwriting questions. This is very valuable, because after the Medigap open enrollment window closes after reaching the age of sixty-five and six months, a question generally asked by Medigap carriers is whether you were eligible for Medicare prior to sixty-five as a result of disability. The implication is clear. If you do not enroll in Medigap at sixty-five, it is unlikely that you will be approved for Medigap under normal medical underwriting.

Disabled and Employer-Sponsored Plan

If you are entitled to Medicare due to non–End Stage Renal Disease (ESRD) disability, Medicare is your primary coverage, if you are not covered by a large employer group plan.[3] If you are covered by an employer-sponsored plan that does not cover at least one hundred employees, Medicare is the primary coverage, and the group plan is secondary.

ESRD and COBRA or Employer-Sponsored Plan

If you have ESRD and any employer-sponsored plan, the employer-sponsored plan is the primary source of insurance for the first thirty months, and Medicare is the secondary payer. After thirty months, Medicare is primary, and the employer-sponsored plan is secondary.

If you have ESRD and COBRA, COBRA is the primary payer for the first thirty months, and Medicare is secondary. It is important to note that the private market (Medicare Advantage or Medigap) is very likely to be superior to a COBRA plan, because the cost and/or coverage is likely to be superior. COBRA usually is another way of saying "overpriced for what you get," and unless it is being paid for by an outside source, it is usually not a good idea to remain under COBRA coverage. Refer to "COBRA Coverage: Should You Take It?" in Chapter 1.

Federal Employee Health Benefits (FEHB)

Eligible persons include both active employees and retirees from the US federal government, including US Postal Service employees and retirees. If you are Medicare eligible you have a couple of difficult choices, and it does depend on whether you are a federal government employee/retiree or a Postal Service employee/retiree.

Enrollment in the FEHB runs on a different calendar than the Medicare Annual Election Period. You can suspend your enrollment in FEHB and reactivate it.[4]

Federal government employees/retirees have access to many variations of comprehensive health and prescription coverage. There is no donut hole in the FEHB program. Further, persons under FEHB can elect an MA/MAPD in addition to their existing benefits, and there is no conflict. In short, it is the same as if a person is entitled to Tricare for Life as described earlier. Even if you stay with the FEHB, you can subscribe to a zero premium MA/MAPD and reap the additional benefits that may be offered with that MA/MAPD plan.

For normal enrollees, FEHB does present an issue, however: price. For federal government employees, the most comprehensive plan is expensive when compared to the private market for similar coverage, except for the donut hole. The bottom line is that if you are in excellent health, it might be prudent to choose a more affordable plan with little or no change in coverage.

Postal Service employees face a different set of circumstances. As of the current writing, the premium charged to Postal Service employees is far lower and cannot be replicated in the private market. For former postal employees, the zero premium MA/MAPD plan, in conjunction with FEHB plan benefits, will result in the lowest cost, along with the additional benefits that can sometimes be offered with MA/MAPD plans.

Spouses of Postal Service employees are charged at different rates from the employee. If the spouse of a Postal employee is Medicare eligible, all of the statements regarding group insurance apply. That may depend upon the Part D coverage gap ("donut hole"); that is, if the spouse of a Postal Service employee/retiree requires many prescriptions, staying inside the FEHB plan may be best.

This Happens

An active Postal Service employee is married to a Medicare-eligible spouse. The spouse elects to not enroll in Medicare Part B when she turns sixty-five. However, over the course of the next year, she develops a medical situation, and her husband retires before turning sixty-five. The human resources representative informs the employee that he and his spouse will no longer be eligible for FEHB benefits. The spouse enrolls in Medicare under a Special Enrollment Period (SEP).

Because she has been ejected from her husband's plan, and since her Part B has not yet become effective, she is able to enroll in Medicare Part B, and elect any Medicare Advantage or Medigap plan available in her location.

State and Local Government Employees

Detroit, Chicago, and Stockton, California, along with countless other locations, face very high legacy obligations, which can result in the bankruptcy of the entire municipality. This can create great uncertainty and turmoil among retirees, while current employees should not blindly assume that retiree benefits are guaranteed.

State government employees could be required to enroll in Medicare Part B when initially eligible, but not necessarily. However, it is highly likely that you will be. Most states describe how Medicare will work with that state's health plan.

Steps to Take

First, you will need to find out if Medicare Part B enrollment is required.

Second, you will need to know how Medicare will work with your employer plan. It is almost always the case that Medicare will be the primary provider, and your state's plan will be secondary because you will be selecting a group Medicare Advantage Plan.

Third, if Medicare is primary and your state's plan is secondary, you will need to find out what your state's plan will cover, beyond what Original Medicare covers. Most plans do not specify whether the Part B Excess charge is paid by the government-sponsored plan. That is another way of saying, "No, but confirm this by yourselves."

Finally, it would be a good idea to find out if you are able to cancel your government-sponsored plan, then reenter at a later date. Again, it is unlikely this would be the case, but you should know this before making a decision.

Local government contracts are usually quite different. Since there can be collective bargaining agreements for certain workers (sanitation, maintenance, transportation), negotitations can be very delicate.[5] Here are some important guidelines.

First, if your local government compensates you for opting out, — that is, pays you cash in exchange for you canceling your group plan — you should examine this carefully. It may well be that this is worth it. If your spouse is not Medicare eligible, he/she can enroll in an individual plan without concern over preexisting conditions, under the Patient Protection and Affordable Care Act (PPACA).

Second, the terms and conditions of your benefits will vary widely from location to location. That will be the single biggest factor in deciding whether you should keep your retiree benefits plan. In the best cases, retiree benefits continue without any changes. In other cases, bankruptcy has been declared, and governments have tried to discontinue retiree health benefits entirely. If you stay in your group plan, the price that will be deducted from your paycheck or pension may be too high. This is especially the case when you figure in the out-of-pocket expenses in conjunction with your group plan and compare it to a Medicare Advantage or Medigap plan.

Third, you need to explore whether you can opt out of your medical and prescription coverage and still retain your dental and vision coverage. You should consider whether the price that you are charged for this dental and vision coverage is worth it, compared to the private market (see "Dental, Vision, and Other Benefits" from Chapter 8).

While it is usually the case that state governments and municipalities are considered to be large employers, this needs to be verified. There can be exceptions in which the actual employer is not a large employer.

Educators

A special type of employee is a public-school educator. Faced with budgetary problems, state governments are being forced to change the benefits packages of both active and retired teachers. The result is that retired teachers have been faced with a changing landscape regarding their retiree health benefits.

In many cases, new teachers will face a future without retiree health benefits. For currently retired teachers, higher premiums may be the result. The point of this is that teachers may need to look at prices, because the price in the private market may soon approach the retiree benefits package's price. The type of group has changed, but the message is the same: educators will not be able to simply presume that their retiree benefits package is the best that they can afford.

Since it is safe to call the statewide educational bodies a "large employer," all the information in Chapter 8 needs to be considered.

UNIONS

Union membership is down nationwide, and this is not news to anyone. This section does not include hourly UAW members, who are covered by the Retiree Benefits Trust, a Voluntary Employees' Beneficiary Association (VEBA) trust. Unfortunately, the bottom line is union retirees will face many of the same things that other Medicare-eligible employees face. Most times, union contracts heavily favor active employees.

Union officials have motivations to promote group plans. One primary reason is that group pricing may be dependent upon the number of enrollees in the retiree group plan, or the percentage of enrollment. While that may be admirable for the group as a whole, the problem is that it may not be good for the individual, i.e., you.

What this means is that if you have a medical situation, you are back to the base case. You need to fend for yourself. Examine for yourself, investigate for yourself, and, ultimately, decide for yourself. Unless the collective bargaining agreement has closed down the Medicare Part D coverage gap, and you or your spouse require medications that exceed Medicare Part D coverage, the almost-inevitable conclusion will be that an individual plan, whether that is a Medicare Advantage or a Medigap policy along with a stand-alone prescription drug plan, will be more cost-effective.

The recommendations made here may seem controversial, because as part of a union, you probably have friends and colleagues who are roughly your age. Those friends or colleagues have gone through the Medicare system. The main piece of advice to leave with you is simple: Your individual situation can be different from your friend's, and do not presume that just because things have "worked out well" that it fits your individual situation. This may seem self-evident, but people reason this way very frequently. In other words, just because your friend jumped off a bridge doesn't necessarily mean that it is a good idea for you.

HOSPITAL (AND OTHER HEALTH-CARE) EMPLOYEES

For personnel who work at hospitals or home health-care services, it is sad and disappointing to report that the health benefits available to retirees of these organizations may be no better than your average group employer in an industry unrelated to health. In fact, health-care organizations frequently discontinue health insurance entirely once a person becomes inactive.

In hospitals, you may know that active employees can work beyond the age of sixty-five. Health-care providers vary widely, so you will need to carefully read to identify your situation.

One special provision can accompany group coverage for hospital employees: prescription drugs are often offered to hospital employees at substantial discounts. These discounts, if combined with the lack of coverage gap, can represent substantially lower out-of-pocket prescription drug expenses.

SMALL BUSINESS OWNERS

At the end of Chapter 8, there is a section called "What Employers Can Do." The issues and challenges stated in that section are ones that should be very familiar to the small business owner. In addition to those issues there are additional challenges that need to be faced, since the business owner is the main stakeholder. There may be legal, tax, and accounting issues, all of which are ultimately the responsibility of the owner.

Depending upon the size and scope of the business, the owner may require an outside advisor. From a health insurance perspective, a Medicare-eligible small business owner should keep a few things in mind.

The new regulations that index your Medicare Part B and Part D premiums to income are complicating matters for high-income earners. It may be that the cost of the premiums is as high as your small business group health insurance premium.

For example, if you make $214,000 a year as a single female, then your monthly Part B premium will be $433.60 a month plus $70.90 a month (Part D IRMAA). When you add a Medigap plan, and a Part D premium, your health insurance total premium can approach or exceed $700 a month. Depending on the state, employer plans may be established that include tax benefits for funds used to pay for premiums and out-of-pocket expenses.

While it may be very possible to find a more economical configuration under a small-employer group plan, caution is required. That is because Medigap Plan G has no cost-sharing provisions after you pay the Medicare Part B deductible. The premiums are your entire medical cost (except for prescriptions).

There may be tax implications to your selection, depending upon the legal structure of your business. You may be taking a business deduction for the cost of health insurance. You should receive tax or financial counseling before deciding on this important matter. In this instance, it may be wise to consult your tax advisor.

One word of warning — some insurance companies will not be able to sell certain Medigap plans if you are opting out of group plans. This is beyond the "normal" restrictions that occur when a person qualifies for a Special Enrollment Period.

PROFESSIONAL "ASSOCIATIONS"

Doctors, lawyers, accountants, dentists, etc. all have professional affiliations of some sort. Within these, there is a decidedly mixed bag. While some organizations are established within a specific state, some are national in scope and scale. There can be associations within a profession, like those for oncologists within the profession of physician. If you belong to such an association and it offers health insurance, you may have been too busy to consider the outside market. You need to consider whether the insurance company that sends you the package deal is doing so as a commercial endeavor.

The bottom line here is that if you live in a state with expensive premiums, the association premium may be lower than the one available to other residents in your geographical location. There is no shortcut to checking this on a case-by-case basis.

This Happens

A professional has been privately insured through his private practice and continues to work through his sixties. He is eligible for and enrolls in Medicare Part A and Part B. In addition, his professional organization offers private health insurance (at group rates), which is more than $300 a month more expensive than Medigap Plan and a stand-alone prescription drug plan (Medicare Part D). It does so without offering or sending out the professional any information regarding Medigap or the cost-sharing arrangement that is available under Medigap. The professional eventually is informed about Medigap and correctly makes the change to Medigap and Part D. It had cost him more than $10,000 in excess premium for coverage that is no better than Medigap and a stand-alone prescription drug plan.

There is no sense in pointing fingers. At this point, $10,000 is gone. It doesn't matter how rich you are, $10,000 is a lot of money that could have been otherwise saved or spent (that may be the least controversial statement in this book). *Maximize Your Medicare* was written so you can do something for yourself that others will not. Even professional associations, created to defend its members, can fall woefully short.

SERIOUSLY ILL

Those who are seriously ill face difficult choices. By seriously ill, I mean that you have a condition that will not improve over time. Even among those persons, there is a very large difference among the types of illness, and as a result, there are different factors to consider.

If you take a lot of medications, you must

choose the best stand-alone prescription drug plan (Part D) that you can afford. While the monthly premiums are higher, these plans are more likely to have lower copays for nongeneric drugs. In addition, many higher-priced plans will have benefits even inside the coverage gap ("donut hole"). Sometimes, patients take a large number of medications but do not require frequent visits to the physician.

Alzheimer's patients may, in certain cases, be in a maintenance mode, where relatively few office visits are required. If that is your situation, then the extra dollar should be used for prescription coverage, and not for medical insurance. If you are choosing a Medicare Advantage Plan, you should recognize that the prescription benefits within different Medicare Advantage Plans can vary, and that can result in a large difference to you.

If you require frequent office visits in order to monitor your situation (for example, type 1 diabetes), your situation is slightly different. You will require frequent examinations (eye exam, foot exam) in order to monitor the disease's progression. In addition, if the situation spins out of control, the complications are serious and could require surgical procedures. For you, the Part B Excess may become an issue, unless you live in a location that disallows charging the Part B Excess, or unless your Medicare Advantage Plan disallows balance billing.

In 2018, the (CHRONIC) Care Act[6] introduced the possibility that social services will be added to Medicare Advantage Plans, to deal with social issues that affect the health and well-being of those with chronic illness. These additional benefits could include home-delivered meals, transportation for nonmedical needs, pest control, indoor air-quality equipment (e.g., air conditioner for someone with asthma), and minor home modifications (e.g., permanent ramps, widening of hallways or doorways to accommodate wheelchairs).[7]

Diabetes

There is no easy way to say it: diabetes has reached epidemic proportions in the United States, with 30.3 million people suffering from some form of it according to the American Diabetes Association. Of Medicare-eligible people in the US, 12.9 million aged sixty-five or older, 25.2 percent had diabetes in 2015. Diabetes is the leading cause of kidney failure, non traumatic lower-limb amputations, and new cases of blindness among adults in the United States.

For people with type 2 diabetes, medications are available, and they are very inexpensive. Generics used to treat diabetes are among the cheapest in the market. As long as things do not spin out of control, it is possible to keep your total health-care costs down.

Type 1 diabetes is treated differently among Medigap carriers. For new applicants, type 1 diabetes can lead to denial by certain carriers, and acceptance by other carriers. Remember that carriers do have the prerogative to make that determination, and their underwriting rules can change. That said, you may have the regulated right if you were leaving a group plan — a certain set of Medigap plans (A, B, K, L) would remain as guaranteed-issue for a period.

For type 1 diabetes patients, prescription coverage is a complicated matter because of the use of insulin. Needles used for insulin injections are defined as durable medical equipment covered by Medicare Part A. Nowadays, insulin is dispensed through a pen, which is part of the prescription. If you are dependent upon insulin, then you will usually reach the Medicare Part D coverage gap ("donut hole"). It may be wise to select a Part D plan that has benefits even when in the coverage gap.

A relatively new development is that a very select number of Medicare Advantage Plans have classified certain types of insulin as generic medications, with copays that are saving diabetics many thousands of dollars a year.

End Stage Renal Disease (ESRD)

End Stage Renal Disease (ESRD) leads to complexity with Medicare. In addition to the very high cost of dialysis, the combination of Medicare, group health insurance, Medicare Advantage, and Medigap is very complicated.

Here are the simple guidelines:

Medigap is available for ESRD patients during Medigap open enrollment.

Medicare Advantage is generally not available for ESRD patients, unless the patient is eligible for Medicare before the age of sixty-five.

Third, if the patient or spouse works, Chapter 7 would be good to review because, depending on the size of the employer, Medicare may be primary or the group health insurance plan may be. For dialysis, the financial difference between the two can be large. The point here is that dialysis is going to be required on a consistent basis, with no end (other than transplant). The cost can be enormous over the long run, and it may be wise to pay a higher premium, if that lowers the total costs (premium plus out-of-pocket expenses).

Conclusions

This chapter may seem to be a list of unrelated groups and unrelated situations. However, they are here to illustrate a single, unified point: under many special circumstances, following the status quo, unchallenged, can be unwise. There is a very long list of reasons that not checking is a decidedly poor decision.

Group health plans for active employees and retirees are changing, with a trend toward much higher deductibles. Professional advisors may not have a full grasp of Medicare. Human resources personnel may not know the developments in the Medicare Advantage market or Medigap.

People you know may be well meaning, but their individual circumstances may not be the same as yours. Here is a partial list of potential differences that may exist between you and someone you know: health situation, financial resources, personal priorities, or marital status. As stated in the

Introduction, a huge challenge facing every person eligible for Medicare is that a single fact can entirely change which Medicare path is best. Hopefully, this incomplete list of groups has raised awareness of this fact.

Chapter 10
The Savvy Medicare Consumer

Truths and Myths

Truth: Medicare is a vital cornerstone of virtually everyone's retirement savings plan.

Truth: Many financial advisers do not understand Medicare, and that leads to you taking unknown financial risks.

Myth: Representatives of insurance companies and agents are all equally able to explain Medicare to everyone.

Stay Focused on the Goal

There is a lot of noise surrounding Medicare. Most of the headlines that predict Medicare's impending doom ignores political reality. That there are sixty million Medicare beneficiaries also means that there are sixty million voters. For Medicare beneficiaries, a single objective remains: obtain the most suitable coverage, at the lowest possible overall costs, to suit your needs today and in the future.

That said, the only logical conclusion is that there will be ongoing changes to the Medicare system. This is due to the fact that ten thousand people turn sixty-five every day in the United States, and Medicare strains the national governmental budget. Headlines appear, every single year, to prove the point.[1] There are changes that can dramatically impact the out-of-pocket costs you will face or your access to health-care services. Carriers adjust to the market in your geographical location, and they make choices to improve or reduce their market share in a specific location.

This is not always negative. For example, networks under Medicare Advantage Plans have improved: Premiums can be $0, and health and prescription drug deductibles can be lower than Medigap and Part D. Competition among Medigap carriers means that premiums can differ by less than $5 a month in many locations, for those turning sixty-five years old. As mentioned in Chapter 4, there are generally between twenty-two and thirty Part D plans available in every location in the nation. While some may believe that there are too many choices, it would be practically impossible to find a "one size fits all" for sixty million

Medicare beneficiaries.

Even though the options are extensive and your consumer rights are well protected, that does not mean that applying for Medicare is trouble-free. Even after you become enrolled in Medicare, there can be issues due to human error or misunderstanding.

Dealing with Medicare Problems

Even people with a great deal of professional experience in complicated business matters, including those involved with health care, can face hurdles when it comes to Medicare. There are many reasons this can occur, and resolving problems can be complicated. This is an incomplete list of problems facing applicants and existing Medicare beneficiaries.

Social Security Administration

This is very scary, but it does occur. Sometimes, you do not exactly describe your situation. Sometimes, a Social Security Administration employee has misunderstood. The reasons do not matter, really. The bottom line is that sometimes you receive the wrong information regarding your Medicare eligibility or when your Medicare coverage begins. There are appeals procedures, which will be covered later in this chapter.

Enrollment Problems

As people work beyond sixty-five, enrollment problems and issues are appearing more frequently. Most of the time, this occurs because the applicant errs in filling out an application or does not have the precise answers that carriers require. Too frequently, people conveniently claim "the insurance company is wrongfully attempting to deny the application." While frustrating, this does not mean that the insurance carrier is violating a federal regulation. Practical reality tells you that it is very unlikely; carriers are highly regulated and require proper documentation before accepting an application.

Cancellation and Reapplying

Cancellation of group plans, whether as an employee or as a retiree, and then applying for a new Medicare Advantage, Medigap, and/ or Part D plan can be very frustrating, and subject to delays. You may be stuck in "no-man's-land," not quite understanding your status. This can be very worrying for the applicant. In this instance, a financial representative with direct access to enrollment departments can be very helpful.

This Happens

A part-time consultant, sixty-eight years old, has been enrolled in health insurance, under COBRA, since December 31, 2018. He considers other employment but decides that Medicare is the best path for himself and his spouse. He correctly completes the government form CMS-L564E and proceeds to the Social Security Administration office during June 2019. He is incorrectly informed by the Social Security employee that he will need to wait until January 2019. However, because he is correctly informed that he has eight months, from January 1, 2019, he firmly asks the Social Security employee to verify this with a supervisor. To his relief, his Medicare eligibility is confirmed with an effective date of August 1, 2019.

In this case, he has been misinformed by the Social Security Administration. This is a scary scenario, because it is completely reasonable to rely on the information from a person employed by the federal government.

There is almost no way that an inexperienced person would have been equipped to defend himself in this situation. Only a person fully confident in the exact rules of Medicare eligibility would have known to be persistent enough to argue with the US government. In this case, a professional's assistance was fully in order. (Yes, it was me.)

Customer Service Departments

In every case, you can call your carrier if you have questions about your coverage or bill. The challenge is that the quality of the information that you receive may vary widely. It would be ideal to report that your questions will be resolved with one phone call. However, that is frequently not the case, for a variety of reasons. While we are not going to settle the issue here, the fact is that insurance carriers may be outsourcing the customer service function to a third party. As a result, that person may not be an expert when it comes to your specific plan in your geographical location.[2]

There can be limits to what a financial representative can do, because certain carriers do not allow direct access to billing departments, while others do allow the representative to speak directly with a qualified person at the insurance company. Agents have special access to insurance companies; that is, they will dial different numbers to ask questions for their clients. If you are the type of person that doesn't like dealing with toll-free numbers and being put on hold, then a qualified agent will be able to help you.

It is very important to keep notes and to keep all written correspondence from your carrier, especially if you encounter problems. The reason is that documentation will be required if you want to file an appeal or grievance. While the process is complicated, it is possible to have denials of coverage overturned, through formal processes.

Appeals

If your health-care service under Medicare Part A or Part B is denied by the CMS, there is a formal appeals process. There are five levels, and it is not easy, nor is it fast. There are expedited appeals possible. In addition, depending on the seriousness of your appeal, there are attorneys that are experienced in this process.

The following are the five levels of the Medicare Part A and Part B appeals process:[3]

- First level: Redetermination by a Medicare Administrative Contractor (MAC)
- Second level: Reconsideration by a

Qualified Independent Contractor (QIC)
- Third level: Decision by the Office of Medicare Hearings and Appeals (OMHA)
- Fourth level: Review by the Medicare Appeals Council
- Fifth level: Judicial Review in Federal District Court

Part D Late Enrollment Penalty Appeal

This process is different. You will be sent a notice from the Part D or Medicare Advantage Prescription Drug Plan carrier, informing you of the Part D Late Enrollment Penalty. You will receive an LEP Reconsideration Notice and an LEP Reconsideration Request Form[4] with the written notification. Note that you will be asked to provide documentation with your appeal form.

Medicare Advantage Appeal

If your service is denied or if your Medicare Advantage Plan carrier refuses to pay your health-care provider, you can file a request for reconsideration directly with the carrier. The carrier will respond within either thirty or sixty days,[5] and if your request is denied, then your request will be automatically elevated to the next level (Level 2). If your

Level 2 reconsideration is denied, then Levels 3 through 5 exist as documented in the same manner as described above. You can request an immediate or expedited review, depending on the urgency of your specific health situation.

Grievances

A grievance is different from an appeal, as defined by Medicare. A grievance can be filed by you against your plan or health-care provider if you are dissatisfied with some aspect of the service that you receive. For example, you may face ongoing billing errors. You may believe that your health-care provider is not providing the quality of care that you believe you need. You can call Medicare directly (800-MEDICARE) to speak with a representative to file a grievance.[6] Medicare Advantage and Part D plans are required to respond to a grievance within thirty days, in writing.

PROFESSIONALS, AMATEURS, AND ADVERTISEMENTS

Do You Need Professional Advice?

Knowing your rights and options is entirely different from *executing* your plan. Filling out applications correctly and answering the questions accurately is a very important step that is frequently overlooked. People are relieved when they understand Medicare enrollment rules, but that is not the actual endpoint. Next is the implementation and the maintenance of your Medicare configuration.

There is a lot of advice out there on what you can or should do. Some of it comes from your employer. Some of it comes from your colleagues at work, your family, or your friends. Sometimes, it will be correct. Unfortunately, that is not always the case. The source of misinformation can even come from official personnel, at governmental agencies or at your workplace.

Opinions on whether you require professional services are everywhere. Senior centers may have volunteers to fulfill this function. Sometimes, these people carefully reveal the limits of their lack of permission to give specific advice, and limits to the information they provide. A volunteer, unless he or she has a license, is not permitted to make recommendations. It takes a specific license to give advice.[7]

Financial representatives could perhaps offer a valuable service. There are many different types of advice you can receive. There is a difference between captive agent and broker. A captive agent is required to tell you the truth; that is undisputed. However, a captive agent does not have the specific permission to be your representative for carriers and plans he/she does not represent. Given that there are important differences in benefits and premiums, a captive agent may not be able to give you the full picture of a very competitive market. A broker may be able to help, but that will depend on the carriers he/she represents.[8]

Remember that Medicare is different in important ways from other health insurance. Insurance agents/brokers that deal with your group plan or financial markets may not have a background in dealing with Medicare. It is important that your agent specifically understands Medicare. The financial stakes are too high, and the first unexpected dollar spent from your savings is likely to be on health care.[9]

Advertisements: Can You Believe Them?

A week may not pass by without you receiving a mailing that promotes a Medicare plan or carrier. Some ads are legitimate, and unfortunately, some are not. Turn on the TV, and you get the same thing — commercials about Medicare are everywhere. This is particularly true at the end of every third quarter, and through the end of each calendar year. Consumer fatigue is understandable, but there are a few things that you must keep in mind.

First, you should keep all mail from the Centers for Medicare & Medicaid Services (CMS) and from the Social Security Administration. It is the official mail from the US government. The Social Security Administration will send you your Medicare card. If you have a Medicare Advantage or Medigap policy, you should keep all statements from the insurance company that has issued the policy to you.

Second, the mail you receive and the advertisements you see, *if sent by Medicare plan carriers,* are not factually wrong. They are highly regulated. In fact, every presentation slide, piece or packet of mail, and advertisement has been specifically approved by the CMS. The conclusion is that it is almost impossible that a mailing you receive, or an advertisement you see on TV, is factually inaccurate, if created by a Medicare Advantage, Part D, or Medigap insurance carrier. If you attend a sales presentation for a Medicare Advantage Plan, then the information on the slides will be accurate; it must be. Even the order of the slides themselves cannot be altered by the presenter.

Third, you should not respond to an advertisement that offers reduced medication prices if you have any type of group health plan that supplements Medicare. Remember, you cannot be enrolled in two prescription plans that are deemed to be creditable coverage by Medicare. This includes the prescription plan that is embedded in a group plan, or an MAPD plan, as long as your prescription benefits program qualifies as creditable coverage. If you mistakenly send in this type of advertisement that enrolls you in a separate Medicare Part D, then the Medicare system will cancel your enrollment in your employer-sponsored group health plan.

This Happens

Mr. Smith is covered by his retiree group plan, including retiree health benefits. He receives a flyer that suggests he can save money on prescriptions, and he sends it in. Three months later, Mr. Smith requires medical attention and presents the insurance card he has used for years. He finds out that the flyer he signed and sent back has enrolled him in a Part D plan, thus dropping the retiree's health benefits plan. Therefore, he is no longer enrolled in that plan and he is then responsible for the costs above the amount that Medicare pays. He only has Original Medicare.

LAST TIPS

The Medicare system isn't perfect, and, so far, our leaders have not come up with plans to improve it and lower health-care costs. Instead, finding solutions to rising health-care costs and maintaining Medicare has evolved into a blame game. The ACA has been blamed, physicians are blamed, pharmaceutical companies are blamed; the list is never-ending. The point of this book is not to assign blame or make judgments about what stakeholder is right or wrong. It is to help you navigate the many twists and turns in the system. Medicare is less complicated than assumed, due to the federally defined enrollment rights and definitions. However, there are many subtleties that depend on your individual situation. You may conclude that you require outside counsel to assist you.

Medicare isn't meant to be comprehensive health insurance. Even if we all agreed on the priorities and politics of the situation, we cannot avoid three fundamental facts:

- There are almost sixty million Medicare beneficiaries, and there are more than ten thousand people turning sixty-five years old every day. They are newly eligible for Medicare, and they live, on average, until eighty years of age. The Medicare-eligible population will only increase over time.

- Pressure on the health-care providers is real. If your child or grandchild dreams of becoming a medical doctor, he/she is looking at $300,000 to $500,000 of educational costs, extraordinary regulatory and legal risk, being a virtual employee of the federal government, and no return on investment at all until he/she is thirty years old (when he/ she starts to pay back debts).
- Payments to hospital systems are under pressure: if Medicare were the only payer to hospital systems, then hospitals, especially those in sparsely populated areas, would be threatened.

Fewer people are paying into the Social Security system, while more people are becoming eligible for Medicare benefits. Now, simply factor in the rising economic pressures on employers, most particularly the rising cost of benefits for active employees. Where will that ultimately leave active employees when they need health benefits, now or in the future? How will employers and employees keep the system going? The only certainty is that the person that will be affected now is you, the Medicare beneficiary.

The choices can be confusing for virtually every segment of the senior population. No one book can possibly cover every scenario, but hopefully this book has given you more knowledge as you enter the Medicare population, so you know what to ask and where to turn.

Remember, verify what you are told. Those giving advice, whether they be friends, agents, or your human resources coordinator, may not have the complete information; they may only know to advise on a limited set of circumstances. In other words, their situation may be different from yours. The things that your friends face, you may not.

Last point: Medicare should be the first stop in retirement planning. The simple reason is that this book reveals that the financial impact of health-care costs can vary widely under Medicare. A single detail can dramatically change your health care and financial outcome in retirement. The difficulty is that Medicare is just one of many moving elements in retirement planning. A combined approach is best, so that the various pieces fit together as a whole. If you do not have the ability to set up such an approach yourself, then a financial planner should be able to do this with you. If your advisor does not have a complete understanding of all of the pieces, find another who understands how best to make all the pieces fit together.

Medicare is the single area where the rights and options are heavily in your favor, if you understand the important health-care and financial implications of the decisions you make. Ultimately, this book is written so that you can take control of your individual situation.

EXPERTS' ADDENDUM

This special section is intended for those with academic backgrounds or practical experience in financial and/or business matters — or the perversely curious.

Insurance Is an Option

In order to understand the conclusions contained in *Maximize Your Medicare,* it is important to understand that insurance is, all things considered, an option, much like a put or a call on a stock. Many people will understand what a put or a call option is, from the financial markets. A simplified version of an option is the refrigerator warranty example presented in the Introduction.

How an option works may be difficult to grasp. An option is the right to buy or sell a product (for example, a stock) for a prespecified price, if a certain set of conditions are met.

The key point is that the value of an option increases rapidly under certain conditions. A call option on a stock increases in value greatly as the underlying stock approaches and exceeds the strike price. In a very similar way, the value of health insurance (including Medicare, Medicare Advantage, and Medigap) also rises dramatically if you incur medical costs, because you receive benefits with significant financial value, which can exceed your premiums by a great deal.

HEALTH INSURANCE IS DIFFERENT

While it is convenient to compare health insurance to auto insurance, dental insurance, or homeowner's insurance, there is a critical difference. Why?

Say you get in a car accident, and you completely wreck your car, but walk away unscathed. What is the cost to you? Do you know? The answer is yes. Open a Kelley Blue Book, and you will be able to determine the salvage value of your car within hundreds of dollars. You can replace your car with an almost-exact copy, at a well-defined price.

On the other hand, imagine that you become seriously ill and are diagnosed with a disease. What are your costs then? Can you predict the price of recovery? You cannot predict when those costs will cease. You cannot predict if you can go back to work to repay those new, unknown costs. Your estimate can be wrong by tens of thousands of dollars. The cost can bankrupt your household, and the outstanding financial liability can leave you in debt for the remainder of your life.

In other words, the benefits from being properly insured with Medicare is immeasurable, but the benefits of owning auto insurance is limited, to the salvage value of your car.

OPTIONS ARE PRICED USING PROBABILITY

Let's get back to the comparison among health insurance, Medicare, and options from financial markets. Options are financial contracts that have a mathematically derived theoretical value. For financial market professionals, this is the widely known Black-Scholes formula. For the purposes of this book, the calculation itself isn't important, but the formula has intuition that we will address here.

Consider "Mistake #1" from the Introduction: the main observation was that health insurance is determined by probability. That is the connection to the Black-Scholes formula, which is also completely dependent on probability. Simply put, most people are familiar with the bell curve. This is what statisticians would call a graph of the standard normal probability curve. Creating this curve requires certain assumptions. An important assumption is that every data point is random and independent; i.e., any previous results do not affect the probability of future results. In theory, that sounds right.

In practice, however, the price of Medicare is cheaper than it should be, given the standard notion of options and how options are priced. Why? Many of the underlying assumptions of the Black-Scholes formula are violated, in your favor, with no effect on the price (premium).

For example, it is not random if you have specific information about your individual circumstance, and you do. Carriers do not know your specific circumstance, but you do. That gives you a definite, distinct advantage, because the carriers cannot change the price of the option when you purchase a Medicare Advantage policy or enroll in Medigap when your acceptance is guaranteed. Your rights are protected by the federal government, and there is nothing that any carrier can do to deny these rights.

The offering price is regulated, you can obtain any Medicare Advantage Plan at the given premium, and, for Medigap, you can purchase it for the best possible price in the market when you turn sixty-five or within six months of enrolling in Medicare Part B.

Let's look at it from the seller's (carrier's) point of view. If you are the seller and you will be required to pay benefits if your customer incurs large medical bills, and the seller knew in advance that high bills will be forthcoming, wouldn't the seller want to charge that customer a higher premium? Of course, the answer is yes. In addition, the future liabilities that the seller could potentially incur are unlimited. Wouldn't you want to charge that customer more?

The obvious answer would be yes, but the fact is that *regulations make this impossible when you first turn sixty years old.* That means that if you, the customer, have a preexisting medical condition or a medical history that makes it very likely that you will require ongoing expensive medical care, the price of Medicare Advantage or Medigap is, if anything, too low. That makes Medicare an option that is very, very inexpensive, compared to the value it will deliver to you.

You don't have to know anything about insurance in order to understand this. Just compare Medicare to the price of health insurance for a sixty-four-year old: high-quality health insurance, which would still be inferior to Medicare, costs more than $1,000 per month.

Everyone Is "Short" an Option

In financial markets, you can benefit, as an investor, if any financial asset goes up or down (that is possible). You can buy or sell an option, a financial contract, that increases in value if the price of gold increases. In addition, you can also buy or sell a set of securities that go up if the price of gold decreases.

In the same way, your household net worth faces the risk of large health-care expenses. The extent of decline has no limit in extreme scenarios. That is very similar to being short an option, much like the investor that is short the price of gold, which is damaging to that investor if the spot price of gold increases. Everyone, irrespective of financial resources, is short this option; i.e., everyone is getting older, and the probability of requiring medical care is increasing with time.

The bottom line: Buying health insurance

is like buying an option at a regulated, highly competitive price, with you being in complete control of your health and financial situation. This is almost never available under any other financially important situation. That option protects your household net worth, because it allows you to not spend your savings/investments at precisely time that you require medical services.

Sources of Volatility

Let's go back to the Black-Scholes formula. The value of a put or a call option increases as volatility increases. In simple terms, that means if there is a wider array of potential outcomes, the shape of the bell curve will be different (but it will be symmetric).

When considering the value of Medicare and health-care cost planning, the volatility increases under a wide variety of situations. Let's take a look at a few, the value of health insurance, and the specific case of Medicare.

Substantial Assets

If you have substantial assets, you can use this method of thinking to understand other conclusions. Since health insurance will continue to pay benefits to the policyholder, irrespective of amount, that means that the wealthier the person is, or the more assets that person has, the more the actual financial value of Medicare or a health insurance contract, from the buyer's point of view, increases. Why is that? You have more to lose (which is the same thing as saying that your volatility is higher). Thus, the contracts protect more and are, therefore, more valuable.

Medical and Family History

Let's say you are a female, and your mother, grandmother, and sisters have been afflicted with breast cancer. Can you say that you are the average case? No. Put another way, this female is subject to a wider variety of outcomes; her volatility of outcomes is higher. The price of health insurance is substantially more valuable to you, and the carriers cannot adjust the selling price to reflect this fact.

Financially Restrained

For those that need to save every dollar, Medicare Advantage has all the advantages listed above, and another important one. Every Medicare Advantage Plan must always include an annual out-of-pocket maximum limit. The value of the option is high, and when coupled with financial assistance or Medicare Advantage Plans with no additional premium, the cost is very, very low.

The bottom line is that health insurance, especially under the Affordable Care Act (if your state participates in Medicaid expansion) and certainly under Medicare, is, if anything, an underpriced way to protect your assets, irrespective of the level of your household net worth.

Comparing Apples to Apples

Much of the confusion regarding Medicare is that there are a wide variety of choices and wide differences in price. Much of the logic and analysis of how to approach Medicare is actually the result of thinking about comparing the options that you enjoy (due to rules of Medicare) and comparing the benefits that you can receive, at a particular price (premium).

Let's take Medigap Plans F and G. If you look at Table 4, you will see they differ in only one regard: the Part B deductible. Under Plan G, the patient/beneficiary is responsible for the Part B deductible. Under Plan F, the carrier will pay for the Part B deductible. If you put the two plans together, then it should be self-evident: Plan F is slightly superior in coverage, since the language is identical in every other respect, *down to the last letter.*

In 2020, the Part B Deductible is $198. If you assume that you go to your primary-care physician twice in a year, then you will likely meet the Part B deductible. This is the way to compare Plan G to Plan F:

> Add $198 to the Plan G annual premium. That will make Plan G precisely equal in every respect to the coverage of Plan F.

It is almost impossible that the Plan F annual premium will be less than Plan G annual premium plus $198.

You will need to decide if the difference in premium is worth it. Since the terms and conditions of coverage are identical after the Part B deductible is met, then the net difference can be considered a convenience tax, because under Plan F, there is no reconciling your payment of the Part B deductible, since the carrier is responsible for everything.

Some people do not want to struggle with billing departments or deal with administrative error. Sometimes these difficulties do not occur. Others value the lower premium more and will deal with the administrative issues, if they do occur. You can continue this process to consider every aspect of benefits that you receive. This is the decision of the consumer and the consumer alone.

Comparing Medicare Advantage Plans to each other is notably more difficult. As stated in Chapter 5, Medicare Advantage is an annual contract, which means the exercise of comparing apples to apples will change every year. It is practically impossible to believe that this situation will cease to exist. Why? The funds from the CMS change every year, and there are multiple competitors (carriers) trying to win more customers (you) every year.

MEDIGAP VS. MEDICARE ADVANTAGE REVISITED

Many say that it is very difficult to determine if Medigap or Medicare Advantage is superior. Earlier in this book, it is stated that the coverage of Medigap is superior because your financial responsibility is very limited (the Part B deductible), and that coverage cannot be changed over time. Further, premium rate increases must be justified via claims of the overall population of policyholders, not on your individual situation. We can use the information from this section to help compare Medigap to Medicare Advantage.

Let's say you have two agreements, and you already know that the language of Agreement 1 will not change through time, but under Agreement 2, the other party can change the language. Let's now compare the prices, and even if the benefits are identical, it should be clear that Agreement 1 is worth more than Agreement 2. In this simple example, Agreement 1 is Medigap, and Agreement 2 is Medicare Advantage.

Remember that you have the unrestricted right to change from Agreement 1 (Medigap) to Agreement 2 (Medicare Advantage), but not vice versa. That is because if you attempt to change from Medicare Advantage to Medigap, carriers can deny your application, and it is largely within their sole discretion. Further, you will be required to wait until the Annual Election Period, because you cannot cancel a Medicare Advantage Plan to enroll in Medigap during the middle of the year (unless you qualify for an SEP as described in Chapter 6). In short, you can see that this option to change would mean that Agreement 1 *should be* more expensive than Agreement 2. A buyer should be willing to pay for the right to change between the two configurations, *if* all else equal.

That is not to say that all else is equal.

For many, the difference in premium is not worth it, because that extra premium may be needed for some other important purpose.

The question is, "Is the difference in premiums worth it?"

It is notable that Medicare Advantage carriers have made this decision far more difficult because the premiums of Medicare Advantage Plans are frequently $0.00/month, and the cost of maintenance resulting from prescription drug costs can be far lower under Medicare Advantage when compared to Medigap. This book certainly does not say that Agreement 1 is superior to Agreement 2, irrespective of price. Price always matters.

Many make a stunning decision: paying *more* for Agreement 2 when compared to Agreement 1. This happens in many locations, where the most expensive Medicare Advantage Plan is selected, instead of Medigap. As you can see by this Addendum, this configuration contradicts the common-sense reasoning used here. The second stunning decision is that people would enroll in Medicare Part A and Part B alone, because that leaves them exposed to unlimited financial costs if extensive health-care services were required. The negatives of

Medicare Advantage are insignificant when compared to the fact that Medicare Advantage must include an maximum out-of-pocket limit (MOOP) every year.

OUR NATIONAL LONG-TERM CARE PROBLEM

Medicare is robust, with excellent consumer rights. However, the United States has no national long-term care strategy. Medicare is not long-term care. How to take care of the growing elderly population has become the proverbial elephant in the room.

Unfortunately, Medicare, or Medicare Advantage and/or Medigap, cannot be considered the same as long-term care for patients. If you require full-time assistance, or if you require a skilled nursing facility care, that is a substantial out-of-pocket expense. The costs can add up quickly, and ultimately, they can bankrupt a household if you require an extended stay in a nursing home. You most likely know someone like this. In a survey published by Genworth in 2018, a semi-private room in a skilled nursing facility costs $7,441 a month. The cost of an assisted living facility costs $4,000 a month, and a home health aide costs $4,195 a month.[1]

Opinions of people vary greatly; some

people abhor the thought of being admitted to a nursing home, and others do not. Even if you have savings, only the very wealthiest Americans can afford to pay the entire cost. If you have no savings, then the government will pay for your care, which creates stresses on the already-stressed Medicaid system. There are no easy answers for a topic that no one wants to discuss.

Insurance-Based Solutions Exist

In the same way the health insurance provides benefits when health-care costs are incurred, there are insurance-based solutions to deal with long-term care needs if you cannot take care of yourself. Since the potential solutions are insurance-based, and insurance is an option, as described at the beginning of this Addendum, then the common-sense conclusion applies: the way to investigate insurance-based solutions is largely the same as explained throughout *Maximize Your Medicare.*

Long-term care insurance, short-term convalescent care, and riders to hospital indemnity plans are three ways that some amounts can be put aside to counter the cost of skilled nursing home facilities.

Long-term care insurance exists to specifically defray the enormous cost of living in a skilled nursing care facility (nursing home). The benefits would cover, depending on policy, the costs incurred to pay for custodial care and/or skilled nursing care, which can occur at home or at a facility. The terms of the policy will dictate exactly which benefits you will be able to collect and under what conditions. Generally, you would need to be unable to fulfill two activities of daily living (ADLs), and this would need to be certified by a physician.

Long-term care insurance (LTCi) has been controversial, for a variety of reasons. Many carriers have decided to stop offering these types of policies entirely. Qualifying for LTCi is decided by the carrier, and anecdotal evidence suggests the standard required to qualify has become more difficult to meet. Finally, the premiums are subject to change.

That has put people in a difficult position. Medicare doesn't cover custodial care and only covers skilled nursing care for a limited period. Traditional, stand-alone LTCi can be expensive. Let's presume, for the moment, that carriers are also aware of this.

For example, carriers are reporting that

their LTCi enrollments are much lower than previous years. They have responded over the past two years with a new product: the combination of universal life insurance and something called a "rider," which adds benefits that would cover custodial care or skilled nursing care, under certain conditions. The number of sellers of this type of insurance contract has expanded rapidly and are briefly explained in the next sections. What's discussed here are general principles only; insurance companies innovate the products rapidly, and new products constantly appear.

LIFE INSURANCE BASICS

This section is devoted to the interaction between health insurance and life insurance. Health insurance provides coverage for morbidity, which is a state of being ill. Life insurance provides coverage for mortality. When you apply for life insurance, insurance companies may ask you to sign a release, which allows them to access your private health information (PHI). Based on your PHI, insurance companies will record their decision with something called the MIB Group, Inc.'s database.

Both life and health insurance companies belong to this member-owned group. If you have applied for life insurance or health insurance in the past and you have been refused, then this information will be revealed each time you try to apply for insurance in the future.

This fact is not well-understood by most, and the ripple effects can result in unintended consequences.

Term life insurance is easy to understand. You pay premiums until a specified expiry date. Once that expiry date passes, you no longer have life insurance. The insurance company may extend the expiry date, at a different price. That price is generally much higher than the one originally paid. There is no cash value established under virtually all term life insurance policies. It is a little-known fact that underwriting (i.e., the approval process) can be more difficult under term life insurance than whole life insurance, and people apply for term-life insurance companies that have very difficult underwriting standards. The problem is that rejection for term-life insurance can reduce the number of possibilities in the future, when applying for other insurance-based solutions.

Whole life insurance is also easy to understand. You pay premiums, and as long you continue to pay, then the death benefit is paid to the beneficiary that you designate. A cash value is often built, which earns an interest rate that may fluctuate over time, depending on financial markets. If you stop paying premiums, then there are options usually available to you, ranging from a paid-up option to the redemption of your cash value. (There can be tax implications to redeeming your cash value, and you should inform yourself of these ramifications beforehand.)

Universal life insurance is a bit more difficult to grasp. It is usually the case that you can adjust the amount of premium that you pay, in order to keep your policy in force. There is medical underwriting involved, and the premiums that exceed the cost of insurance may build cash value, which can earn returns based on financial markets or fixed interest rates.

Universal life insurance pays a benefit to your beneficiary when you pass away. The premiums will vary, depending on your age, health, biological sex, and financial markets. You can choose to pay more or less and still keep your policy in force.

LIFE INSURANCE AND LIVING BENEFITS

Carriers have added living benefits to life insurance, which generally allow the insured person to use the benefits *in advance,* if certain criteria are met. For example, if you cannot perform two ADLs or if you have been diagnosed with a terminal condition that will require skilled nursing care, then extended benefits may allow you to collect the benefits, and use those benefits to pay for custodial care or skilled nursing care. If the entire death benefit is not completely used, then it is frequently the case that the remainder is paid to your beneficiary/beneficiaries. This has existed in combination with universal life insurance for many years. Recently, this same type of benefit is available in a limited set of term life insurance policies.

If this sounds complicated, it is. There are a number of reasons that contacting an expert would be in order. Just like standalone LTCi, the fine print regarding the criteria that must be fulfilled in order to receive benefits varies among carriers. In addition, there may be tax implications, depending on the amount of benefits received. After advising a wide variety of Medicare beneficiaries, I have been challenged to distinguish among a dizzying number of options.

Most important, the purchase of any interest in any financial contract (and life insurance is a financial contract) must be appropriate for your individual financial situation. For example, a Certified Financial Planner™ would need to fulfill a fiduciary duty to you, which means that he/she would be prohibited from making a financial recommendation if it did not fit your situation.

Annuity-Based Solutions

There are annuity-based solutions. For example, recent innovations allow those that require skilled nursing facility care to receive additional annuity payments. The main principle here is that products are changing, and carriers are innovating continuously in order to address an obvious need.

These Options Are Difficult to Analyze

You may have determined that you can make Medicare decisions by yourself. However, the items described in this Addendum almost certainly require an expert. There are reasons for this. First, and foremost, is that the definitions of the terms and conditions in these contracts is not standardized at all. Carriers can define terms and conditions without federal regulation. That does not mean that carriers will violate the terms and conditions. Nevertheless, it does mean that understanding the implications of these terms and conditions is very difficult. Even more challenging is the task of comparing the many alternatives. Second, the market is changing so rapidly that by the time you have read this addendum, it is a certainty that new developments and new competitors have appeared.

GLOSSARY

Activities of Daily Living (ADLs): There are six ADLs: eating, bathing, dressing, toileting, transferring (walking), and continence. Long-term care insurance may cover a patient if it is documented that he/she cannot conduct three ADLs.

Advance Beneficiary Notice of Noncoverage (ABN): Form CMS-R-131 is issued by providers (including independent laboratories, home health agencies, and hospices), physicians, practitioners, and suppliers to Original Medicare (fee for service, or FFS) beneficiaries in situations where Medicare payment is expected to be denied.

Annual Election Period (AEP): Also known as the Annual Coordinated Election Period. In 2018, the Annual Election Period (AEP) ran from October 15, 2018 through December 7, 2018. Medicare Advantage and Medicare Part D plans can be changed, without restriction, during this time.

Appeal: An appeal is the action you can take if you disagree with a coverage or payment decision made by Medicare, your Medicare health plan, or your Medicare Prescription Drug Plan.

Assignment of Benefits: The compensation given by the Medicare system to a medical provider. Under a PFFS (Private Fee-for-Service), the medical provider must accept Medicare's Assignment of Benefits on a case-by-case basis. Failure by the medical provider to accept the Assignment of Benefits within a PFFS structure will result in no benefits paid from either Medicare or the PFFS plan.

Coinsurance: A percentage of administered services that you, the insured, must pay. For example, if the coinsurance percentage is 20 percent, then your insurance policy will pay for 80 percent, and you are responsible for 20 percent.

Copay: A fixed dollar amount that you must pay. For example, stand-alone Part D plans have fixed amounts that you, the insured, must pay, for a given medication. Medicare Advantage Plans can have copays for health-care services received.

Cost sharing: The combination of deductibles, coinsurance, and copays under a Medicare Part D, Medicare Advantage, or Medigap plan.

Coverage gap: Otherwise known as the "donut hole." For 2020, this begins when your total out-of-pocket expenses (deductible plus copays) reach $4,020 and lasts until your total out-of-pocket expenses reach $6,350.

Creditable coverage: The term is used to describe prescription drug plans. If you have creditable coverage, there will be a certificate, or a page, in your "Summary of Benefits" that describes your group plan. That certifies that your plan meets certain criteria established by the CMS. If you discontinue coverage (either voluntary or involuntary) under a plan that qualifies as creditable coverage, then you may return to Original Medicare or select Medicare Advantage or Medigap under a Special Enrollment Period (SEP). In addition, you can also select a stand-alone Prescription Drug Plan (Medicare Part D). If your plan loses creditable-coverage status, then you will have another SEP, and you are entitled to all changes under SEP privileges.

Custodial care: Care related to Activities of Daily Living (ADLs). Note that this is *not* the same as Skilled Nursing Care. Therefore, it is not covered by Original Medicare. Custodial care is not covered by Medicare Advantage Plans or Medigap plans.

Deductible: A fixed-dollar amount that you must pay *before you receive insurance benefits.* This is subject to change by Medicare or your insurance company. The easy way to remember deductible is that *you are first in line* to pay bills up to the deductible amount.

Durable Medical Equipment (DME): DME is covered by Medicare Part A, with cost sharing. Medicare Advantage and Medigap plans have cost-sharing arrangements that depend on the plan. Needles for insulin injection are part of DME.

End Stage Renal Disease (ESRD): Kidney failure that requires dialysis or transplant. Kidney failure that is not ESRD can occur. ESRD is a specific condition with a percentage failure rate, which must be documented for Medicare purposes and VA benefits purposes. ESRD patients can purchase a Medigap policy but are generally not allowed to purchase a Medicare Advantage (MA) Plan.

Extra Help program: Federal program that offers financial assistance to those that qualify, to defray prescription costs, including Part D premiums, deductibles, and copays. Extra Help beneficiaries can change their prescription drug plan once per quarter during the first three quarters, and during the Annual Election Period. Qualification status can be changed by the Social Security Administration (SSA).

Formulary: A list of approved drugs issued by insurance companies. A formulary can change throughout the year, with restrictions imposed by the CMS. Every medical condition must have at least two medications in its formulary suitable for use, as determined by the CMS.

General Enrollment Period (Medicare General Enrollment Period): This period is no longer available. It has been replaced by the Open Enrollment Period.

Grievance: The action you can take if you disagree with a coverage or payment decision made by Medicare, your Medicare health plan, or your Medicare Prescription Drug Plan.

Health Maintenance Organization (HMO): An organization that provides medical services via contract with member medical providers and facilities. A primary-care physician (PCP) must be selected by the policyholder, and future consultations are approved via referral. If services are received from physicians or facilities, then the HMO will not provide benefits.

Health Maintenance Organization Point of Service (HMO-POS): A type of Medicare Advantage Plan that has a primary-care physician that coordinates in-network referrals. Services received from in-network providers are coded, billed, and coordinated by the PCP. Referrals outside the network are allowed, although the cost-sharing arrangement may not be for full payment of services.

Health Savings Account (HSA): A bank account that can best be considered a "Health Expense IRA." In order to open an HSA, you must be enrolled in a High Deductible Health Plan (HDHP). Funds in an HSA can be used to pay for allowable medical expenses, as defined by the US Internal Revenue Service.

Home Health Care: Home health-care services are offered by privately run agencies, sometimes in conjunction with skilled nursing care facilities. Patients receive custodial care at their home on an hourly or daily basis. Medicare does not cover any costs associated with home health care unless you are under a plan of care established and reviewed by a doctor; you are unable to leave home without considerable effort; and a physician certifies that you require skilled nursing, physical, or occupational therapy, or speech pathology services. The home health agency caring for you must be Medicare certified. The combined services are limited to thirty-five hours per week. The official Medicare description of services is available online: www.medicare.gov/Pubs/pdf/10969-Medicare-and-Home-Health-Care.pdf.

Income Related Monthly Adjustment Amount (IRMAA): IRMAA is an additional amount added to the monthly Part B and Part D premiums for individuals whose modified adjusted gross income (or MAGI) exceeds certain threshold amounts that can change each year. Part D IRMAA is administered by the Part D carrier.

Initial Coverage Election Period (ICEP): A one-time event when a beneficiary can enroll in a Medicare Advantage Plan. It ends the day before a person is eligible for both Medicare Part A and Part B, for the first time, or the last date of the individual's Part B initial enrollment period. You can enroll in a Medicare Advantage Plan only once during the ICEP. You cannot change from plan to plan during this period.

Initial Enrollment Period (IEP): A seven-month period when most people can first enroll in Medicare Part B and Medicare Part D, beginning three months prior to the first date a beneficiary can be eligible for Medicare Part B and Medicare Part D, and ending three months after the last date of the month a beneficiary can be eligible for Medicare Part B and Medicare Part D.

Long-Term Care insurance (LTCi): Insurance that is used to defray costs when the beneficiary cannot perform three ADLs (Activities of Daily Living).

Low Income Subsidy (LIS): See Extra Help program.

Medical Loss Ratio: The Affordable Care Act (ACA) mandates that 80 to 85 percent of all premiums received must be paid to policyholders via claims. If this ratio is not met, then rebates are provided to policyholders.

Medicare Advantage: Plans that are certified by the CMS on an annual basis. They are subject to enrollment rules, with exceptions, called Special Enrollment Periods. They could include prescription drug benefits, but not necessarily. Restrictions may apply with respect to medical provider. Cost-sharing terms and conditions are subject to change on an annual basis with the approval of the CMS. These plans must be, on average, superior to Original Medicare. That does not mean that each specific benefit in a specific Medicare Advantage Plan must be superior to Original Medicare. It means that the plan must be, on average, superior to Original Medicare.

Medicare Advantage Disenrollment Period: January 1 through February 14. This period has now been replaced by the Open Enrollment Period. See *Open Enrollment Period.*

Medicare Advantage Plan: A Medicare health plan offered by insurance companies that are contracted with Medicare. The insurance company administers all aspects of benefits, billing, and your costs. Many Medicare Advantage Plans include prescription drug benefits.

Medicare Advantage Prescription Drug (MAPD plan): A type of Medicare Advantage Plan. It combines hospital insurance, health insurance, and prescription drug benefits. It cannot be used with a standalone prescription drug plan (PDP, also known as Part D).

Medicare-approved amount: The amount Medicare will compensate a medical provider for Medicare Part B services. A prescribed amount, it is also called the Allowed Charge. Any amount above the Allowed Charge is called an excess charge.

Medicare Part A: Hospital insurance as defined by the Centers for Medicare & Medicaid Services (CMS). Includes skilled nursing facility care, home health care, and hospice services.

Medicare Part B: Medical insurance as defined by the Centers for Medicare & Medicaid Services (CMS). Includes services administered by physicians.

Medicare Part C: Also known as Medicare Advantage (MA). Medicare Advantage Plans that include prescription drug benefits are called Medicare Advantage Prescription Drug Plans (MAPD). Medicare Advantage Plans include HMOs, PPOs, PFFS, POS, and HMO-SNPs. Medicare Advantage Plans replace Original Medicare, and insurance carriers process claims.

Medicare Part D: Also known as stand-alone prescription drug plans (PDP). Beneficiaries cannot have prescription coverage from two sources. Prescription coverage is subject to a plan formulary. Can be changed annually without restriction during the Annual Election Period (AEP).

Medicare Savings Programs: There are four Medicare Savings Programs: QMB, SLMB, QI, and QWDI. They are federally funded programs administered by each individual state. These programs are for people with limited income and resources and help pay some or all of their Medicare premiums, deductibles, copayments, and coinsurance. Each state individually applies its specific standards to determine eligibility. A screening tool is available online, Benefit Eligibility Screening Tool (BEST): www.ssabest.benefits.gov/. You can also contact your state Medicaid program to apply.

Medicare Summary Notice (MSN): If you have received Part A or Part B services within the past three months, then you will receive an MSN once every three months. If you have not received any services, then you will not receive an MSN. The MSN will detail the services and amounts that your health-care provider has billed Medicare, what Medicare paid, and the maximum amount that you may owe. It is not a bill.

Medigap: Also known as Medicare Supplement or Medicare Supplemental Insurance. Plans are labeled with letters A through N. The terms and conditions of every plan are standardized among carriers and will remain in effect, unchanged, as long as the policyholder continues to make premium payments.

Military disability: Complicated system that requires a separate application process from Social Security disability. Partial disability categorization is possible. VA-supplied medical insurance and prescription benefits available.

National Provider Identifier (NPI): This is the unique identifier for health-care providers. Medicare Advantage Plans that are HMOs will require the assignment of a primary-care physician, to be identified via his or her NPI.

NOTICE Act: The formal name is the Notice of Observation Treatment and Implication for Care Eligibility Act. The NOTICE Act requires the hospital to inform a patient whether he/she status in a hospital is outpatient (observation) or inpatient.

Open Enrollment Period: This is the reintroduction of the period that begins on January 1 and ends on March 31. During this time frame, an existing Medicare Advantage policyholder can a) switch among Medicare Advantage Plans, and b) cancel enrollment in Medicare Advantage, return to Original Medicare, and enroll in a stand-alone prescription drug plan (Part D). In addition, a person can enroll in Medicare Part A and Medicare Part B, with coverage to begin on July 1 of that year.

Original Medicare: Medicare Part A and Medicare Part B, in combination, are called Original Medicare.

Preferred Provider Organization (PPO): A type of Medicare Advantage Plan that allows participants to receive services from in-network and out-of-network providers. The number of member providers in a PPO is usually larger than the number of member providers in an HMO, thereby allowing for greater freedom of choice in selecting physicians and facilities. Services received from out-of-network providers have costlier cost-sharing terms and conditions than services received from in-network providers. Annual out-of-pocket maximums will be higher if services from out-of-network providers are received.

Primary-care physician (PCP): The physician that you identify if you select a Medicare Advantage HMO. Your PCP must provide a referral if you require services from a specialist.

Private Fee-for-Service (PFFS): A type of Medicare Advantage Plan that requires case-by-case approval by the medical provider. The medical provider must agree to accept the Medicare-allowed charge as full payment. A PFFS is the only Medicare Advantage Plan that allows a Medicare beneficiary to also enroll in a stand-alone prescription drug plan (Medicare Part D).

Short-term convalescent care insurance: Insurance that can be purchased to provide benefits for skilled nursing home care and, in certain cases, custodial care. Beneficiaries can choose whether or not benefits will include custodial care at his or her home. Limitations exist on the length of time that benefits can be received by the beneficiary.

Skilled nursing care: This is a defined term by Medicare. Services must be ordered by a physician and delivered by a registered nurse (RN), who is also a licensed practical nurse (LPN). Services must be deemed to be reasonable and necessary for the treatment of illness or injury.

Skilled nursing care facility (SNF): Also known as a nursing home. A facility that delivers skilled nursing care. Costs are covered by Medicare Part A only after being admitted inpatient at a hospital for at least three days. Long-Term Care insurance can be used to defray costs incurred at a skilled nursing care facility.

Social Security Administration (SSA): Governmental agency that determines Medicare eligibility and Extra Help program qualification.

Social Security Disability Insurance and Supplemental Security Income (SSDI): Benefits paid to those that require assistance due to disability. Applications for these benefits are difficult to obtain, and legal representation is usually required. Those who receive SSDI benefits for twenty-four months are entitled to enroll in Medicare, effective the first day of the twenty-fifth month.

Special Enrollment Period: There are Special Enrollment Periods (SEPs), in which you can either return to Original Medicare or enroll in a Medicare Advantage (MA) plan. In addition, you can appeal for an SEP as well, if the situation does not fit any of the predetermined categories. A description of the SEPs is listed in Chapter 4. There are additional SEPs that can occur due to natural disasters or extenuating situations.

"Summary of Benefits": Document that details cost sharing details with a health insurance policy. You should either receive one annually or be able to request this from your insurance company and/or human resources coordinator at an employer. Details will include terms and conditions of enrollment rules, cancellation rules, deductibles, copayments, and premiums. You should keep the most recent copy for reference.

Term life insurance: Life insurance that pays a death benefit to the named beneficiary upon the death of the insured, as long as the date of death occurs before or on the date of expiry. If the insured survives beyond the date of expiry, then the insurance ends, and the insured becomes uncovered. There is usually no cash value associated with term life insurance.

Whole (Permanent) Life Insurance: Life insurance that pays a death benefit to the named beneficiary upon the death of the insured. Coverage does not expire, regardless of attained age of the insured. Premiums may vary, depending upon the terms and conditions of the policy. Whole Life Insurance may build cash value, which may accrete based on investment performance.

ENDNOTES

Introduction

1 2019 Medicare Trustees Report.

2 Almost all financial contracts, from dental insurance to Medigap, are priced using some modified form of this single formula.

3 While the auto mechanic may be an expert in auto stocks, the mechanic's expertise in the workings of a car's transmission does not specifically qualify him or her to be an expert in auto stocks.

Chapter 1

1 Example: if your claim for SSDI benefits begins on June 1, 2019, there is a five-month waiting period, and from that date, you begin to receive SSDI benefits. From October 1, 2019, you begin to receive benefits. And after receiving SSDI benefits for twenty-four months, you are then

eligible for Medicare Parts A and B on October 1, 2021.

2 For example, there is no such thing as partial Social Security disability, as there is under the rules established by the Veterans Administration.

3 These examples are not meant to be exhaustive; they are illustrations.

4 This penalty is not frequently encountered, but if someone is covered by a large employer and then retires, it could apply, if the person has not enrolled in Part A when turning sixty-five.

5 There is an appeals process, which is administered by a third party.

6 This is an example of the term "adverse selection."

7 This can be found online: www.cms.gov/medicare/eligibility-and-enrollment/origmedicarepartabeligenrol/index.html. It is the case that if your group coverage is cancelled during your IEP, the rules of IEP will determine when Part B coverage begins, and that includes the delays as stated in the section "Timing."

8 If you qualify as a QMB, SLMB, or QI, then all late enrollment penalties are waived.

Chapter 2

1 Quarters of Coverage is the technical term for the ten years. The ten years times four quarters per year equals forty (10 years × 4 quarters per year = 40). Quarters of Coverage is required in order to qualify for Medicare Part A without premium.

2 Table 1 at the end of this chapter will change over time; the most updated version will be available online at www.maximizeyourmedicare.com.

3 Strictly speaking, the benefit period expires sixty calendar days after discharge from the hospital for that particular medical issue. If you have a different medical problem that requires hospitalization, that is another benefit period.

4 The national average for a semiprivate room in a nursing home is $86,764 per year, according to the US Department of Health and Human Services, National Clearinghouse for Long-Term Care Information, October 2017.

5 This is the source of controversy: Medigap carriers cannot alter this, but Medicare Advantage carriers can impose this standard.

6 The complete language of the law can be found online at www.congress.gov/bill/

114th-congress/house-bill/876/text. Hospital systems had to comply with this law by August 6, 2016. This is an important development because patients have not been aware of their status while being treated in a hospital, but this new law makes it mandatory for the hospital to reveal that status and notify the patient in writing. As of this writing, the law is too new to collect evidence that proves whether this statute has been effective.

Chapter 3

1 These tables are found on the book website: www.maximizeyourmedicare.com. They can also be found on www.medicare.gov and many other sites. These amounts are known as the Income Related Monthly Adjustment Amounts (IRMAA).
2 A little-known fact is that funds in an HSA (Health Savings Account) can be used to pay for your Medicare Part B premium. Those people that have saved money in an HSA will likely want to receive a bill, so that they can write a physical check or transmit via electronic transfer to pay for the Part B premium.
3 Part B Excess is explained later in this chapter.

4 The list of services can be found online at www.medicare.gov/coverage/is-your-test-item-or-service-covered.

5 Home health services are described in the Glossary. There are a variety of very complicated conditions required to receive Medicare benefits, which are frequently misunderstood by home health-care service agencies.

6 That is not to suggest that a Medicare Advantage carrier is inferior, because there may be additional benefits, or lower costs, in other areas.

7 This is made more complicated by the fact that a Medicare Advantage carrier may cover the consultation, while a Medigap carrier will not cover a consultation that is not covered by the CMS.

8 www.medicare.gov/coverage/clinical-laboratory-tests.

9 For Medicare Advantage Plan policyholders, there is an official notice called the Integrated Denial Notice, which will detail if your coverage is being denied, discontinued, or curtailed.

10 This is called Medicare assignment. What is one way of asking a health-care provider? "Do you accept Medicare assignment as full payment?"

Chapter 4

1 In Chapter 1 and Chapter 9, there are additional sections which describe being eligible for Part D coverage prior to the age of 65, including when the Part D Late Enrollment Penalty begins prior to the age of sixty-five. The Part D Late Enrollment Penalty is separate from the Part A and Part B Late Enrollment Penalties.

2 If you qualify for the federal Extra Help program, then the Part D Late Enrollment Penalty is waived. However, if you were to lose Extra Help eligibility in the future, then the Part D Late Enrollment Penalty would resume from the date that your Extra Help coverage ends.

3 If you are enrolled in a Medicare Advantage Prescription Drug Plan, then IRMAA will be added to the stated MAPD premium.

4 This is a very large increase from 2019, when the catastrophic coverage stage began at $5,100.

5 According to the Medicare Payment Advisory Commission (MedPAC) in its report dated March 2019, thirty-three thousand beneficiaries filled a prescription that was expensive enough to place them in the program's catastrophic phase after

a single claim in 2010. By 2016, that number had risen to 360,000.

6 There have been proposals to discontinue the discount from pharmaceuticals within the coverage gap, which is a huge problem for those that have expensive brand-name medications.

7 Very important note: you can sort by Lowest Estimated Annual Mail Order Costs, in addition to Lowest Estimated Annual Retail Costs. The answers can be different; do not assume that the order will be the same. In fact, it is very likely that the order will change when you sort differently.

8 If you know that you will be in a different geographical location, or if you travel frequently, then selecting a nationally available pharmacy in multiple locations may affect the decision of the most efficient Part D plan.

9 2019 update: The combination of preferred pharmacies and formularies, along with the plan, continues to make selection much more difficult than it appears. While the average plan in 2019 has a lower monthly premium, the difference in total prescription drug expenses will vary widely, based on the specific pharmacies that a person prefers. If the pharmacy is

not a preferred pharmacy, then the total prescription cost can be much higher under that plan.

10 Kaiser Family Foundation, "Key Findings from the Kaiser Family Foundation 2012 National Survey of Seniors: Seniors' Knowledge and Experience with Medicare's Open Enrollment Period and Choosing a Plan," October 2012, http://www.kff.org/medicare/issue-brief/seniors-knowledge-and-experience-with-medicares-open/.

11 Social Security Administration, "Understanding the Extra Help with Your Medicare Prescription Drug Plan," https://www.ssa.gov/pubs/ EN-05-10508.pdf.

Chapter 5

1 Medicare Payment Advisory Commission, "Report to the Congress: Medicare Payment Policy," March 2019. When the words "on average" are used, this relates to the term "actuarial equivalence." While the overall Medicare Advantage Plan must meet or exceed the average terms and conditions of original Medicare, specific clauses can differ from the coverage described in Chapters 2 and 3.

2 This is quite different from individual

health insurance, or an HMO provided by an employer. In those instances, a referral is usually required.

3 It is clear that Medicare Advantage Plan sponsors (insurance companies) have intentionally allocated this segment of Medicare beneficiaries, by providing additional benefits that may not exist in Medicare Advantage Prescription Drug Plans.

4 There are exceptions. See Chapter 6, "State-Specific Medigap Rights." In New York and Connecticut, this is the period when a person can cancel his or her Medicare Advantage policy, select a Part D plan, and enroll in Medigap. The applicant can do so because there are no underwriting requirements for acceptance.

5 A prime example is that the CMS extended the Annual Election Periods for those affected by the effects of hurricanes and disruption caused by the wildfires in California. In this instance, evidence must be provided that you qualify. Another example is if the Medicare Advantage Plan is canceled by the CMS due to financial difficulties at the carrier.

6 For those that have other creditable prescription drug coverage and do not wish to include prescription drug benefits

within the Medicare Advantage Plan, the third selection, Medicare Health Plans without Drug Coverage" should be selected.

7 If there are questions, you can call the carrier directly. While infrequent, errors do exist on an insurance company's website.

8 This poses challenges, since the CMS has reported that it found a high error rate in its Online Provider Directory Review Report at www.cms.gov/Medicare/Health-Plans/ManagedCareMarketing/Downloads/Provider_Directory_Review_Industry_Report_Round_3_11-28-2018.pdf.

Chapter 6

1 The word "supplement" has been misused by retiree group-plan sponsors. Medigap is a very specific term that refers to the specific plans described in this chapter. To state that an employer-sponsored group retiree health plan "supplements" original Medicare is not the same as being covered by Medigap.

2 While the Medigap open enrollment period lasts for six months from the first date of Part B coverage, the Part D enrollment rules still apply as stated in Chapter

4. For our John Smith, the last day to enroll in Part D is June 30, 2016, regardless of the date that he applies for a Medigap policy.

3 States may also have additional, expanded rights to apply for Medigap. These are the minimum standards.

4 This is the most subtle of options. For example, you can intentionally switch temporarily to Medicare Advantage, for the sole reason of obtaining Guaranteed Issue to Medigap at a lower premium level.

5 Note that these are examples, and the carriers or states have the discretion to change these expanded paths over time, since they are not federally mandated. An expert is required, since the carrier and location will vary from state to state, from situation to situation, and from carrier to carrier. There is no way around this. A special word of caution is that many agents will not be fully aware of the subtleties stated in this section.

6 If you attempt to enroll in Medigap yourself, you need to make very careful note of which exact term is being used by the carrier.

7 There is no universally accepted terminology for this among carriers. The word

"simplified" was selected to describe the catch-all category where Medigap open enrollment and Guaranteed Issue rules do not apply.

8 Please refer to Table 4. Plans K and L differ slightly in their coverage from all other plans.

9 The $176 per day copay for days twenty-one through one hundred is reset annually, so the daily charge may be larger over time.

10 The exceptions are Plans C and F, which are closed to new applicants beginning on January 1, 2020. Existing policyholders are not responsible for the Part B deductible.

11 The copay is refunded to you if you are admitted to the hospital, because then your coverage would be provided under Medicare Part A.

12 Some anticipate future premium changes, based on the fact that Plans C and F will be discontinued for new applicants, beginning on January 1, 2020. However, that assumes that subdividing groups of policyholders does not occur today. That assumption is incorrect: carriers frequently redefine "risk pools" of policyholders over time.

13 As my extensive experience in analyzing

financial contracts for commercial and private use attests, it is not an understatement: Medigap is one of the best, if not the very best, financial contract in favor of the buyer. The terms and conditions are universally understood by competing carriers and health-care providers, since they must adhere to federally defined (albeit confusing) terms.

14 "Catastrophic" is entirely dependent on household net worth. By "superior," the point is that Medigap's language, its terms and conditions, are superior. Both Medicare Advantage and Medigap prevent catastrophic financial losses because there is a cap on maximum out-of-pocket expenses, which Medicare Part A and Part B alone do not provide.

15 The provisions of the ACA against excluding preexisting conditions do not apply to Medigap; the ACA refers to primary coverage. Medigap is secondary coverage.

16 The list of additional benefits is definitely going to grow as the CMS has included meal delivery and air-conditioning units as services or equipment that can improve the health of Medicare Advantage policyholders.

17 While it is impossible to state precisely

why the market share of Medicare Advantage policyholders has grown, the intuition is clear: people have begun to become educated and decided that the overall benefits of Medicare Advantage satisfy their personal requirements. This list presents just a few of the reasons our clients have chosen Medicare Advantage, and we have supported their private decisions.

18 For example, some carriers are now offering health-club memberships to policyholders.

19 For example, certain carriers have added health-club discounts, and the intense price competition may result in meaningfully lower premiums, depending on the carrier and your geographical location.

20 For those that do have federally protected rights, there is no need to worry. This section is for those that want to enroll in Medigap after federal protections have expired, and if carriers in your location do not offer guaranteed acceptance provisions.

21 Insurance companies must justify rate increases by proving a Medical Loss Ratio (MLR). In fact, as of August 2012, insurance companies have been required to issue refunds if claims did not represent a ratio of premiums (less regulatory costs).

The idea that carriers can randomly increase premiums is incorrect.

22 Per the Medicare Access and CHIP Reauthorization Act of 2015. Carriers are making certain exceptions for existing Medigap policyholders, depending on the state.

23 The exception is if the carrier itself ceases to exist due to bankruptcy. However, even in that instance, a Special Enrollment Period (SEP) is almost certain.

24 If you have had health insurance continuously for the six months prior to Medicare eligibility, then no insurance company can deny you coverage under this stipulation. Depending on the carrier, you may be asked to provide evidence that you were covered by health insurance during the prior six months.

Chapter 7

1 Commonwealth Fund, https://www.commonwealthfund.org/. May 23, 2019.

2 As long as the prescription drug benefits are deemed to be creditable coverage by the CMS.

3 Please refer to the section "Can I Delay My Enrollment in Medicare?" in Chapter

1, "Enrollment."

4 Spouse and dependents will have the right, but not the obligation, to enroll in an ACA-compliant plan under a Qualifying Life Event, because they will lose their coverage under the employer-sponsored plan.

5 For example, there are little-known plans that are very similar to Medigap coverage, available for employees and retirees.

6 That does not mean that an employee would always exit employer-sponsored coverage. For example, if the spouse or dependent had no other affordable access to health insurance, even after considering Medicaid expansion states with premium subsidy, then the only logical choice may be to remain with small employer group-sponsored coverage.

7 The ACA has definitely resulted in a wider set of options for the spouses and dependents of employees, because they will qualify for a Qualifying Life Event under ACA rules. Depending on the household's financial situation, the spouse and/or dependents may also qualify for a premium tax subsidy and/or cost-sharing advantages.

8 There are an almost endless number of combinations. This is not meant to be a

complete list. Rather, it points out factors that can make a very large financial impact, improve benefits, or both.

9 This will depend on the state in which you live. Not all states have adopted Medicaid expansion. Some states have state-specific assistance programs.

10 This can be found online: www.cms.gov/medicare/CMS-Forms/CMS-Forms/Downloads/CMS-L564E.pdf.

Chapter 8

1 The list of employers that have either gone bankrupt or reduced retiree health benefits greatly is too long to detail here.

2 The Supreme Court has ruled that retiree health benefits are not guaranteed in the same way that pension benefits are, unless explicitly documented.

3 For certain retirees, this is a tragedy, since contributions were not made via the Social Security Administration, and those retirees do not qualify for Medicare Part A. They would need to pay.

4 In a very subtle difference from the ACA, a small employer is defined as having fewer than fifty eligible employees, which is calculated by the addition of full-time employees, plus the number of hours

worked by part-time employees.

5 It is not difficult to predict that both small and large employers will be using the new structures due to the increasing number of people that work beyond sixty-five.

6 You will need to check with your human resources contact and ascertain whether you must enroll in Part B in order to qualify for retiree health benefits from a large employer.

7 Anecdotal evidence suggests employers do not allow you to "change your mind" and revert back to employer-provided retiree health benefits plans. The notable exception is the Federal Employee Health Benefits (FEHB) program, under which you can suspend your benefits and then revert back in the future.

8 This is not all bad news. In fact, for certain Medicare Advantage carriers, the Medicare Advantage definition of "in network" is superior to the pre-Medicare definition.

9 Some large employers do allow you to retain your dental and vision benefits and cancel your retiree health benefits. There is no rule here, so you will need to check the employer's policy on this. To make matters more difficult, the working policy of the employer is subject to change; there

is no regulation that protects you from a change in your employer's working policy.

10 Certain employers are effectively paying active employees for canceling their employer-sponsored health insurance plans. Note that the proposed Medicare for America has elements that closely resemble this.

Chapter 9

1 This section assumes that a veteran knows how to register in the Defense Enrollment Eligibility Reporting System, otherwise known as DEERS (www.tricare.mil) or the Department of Veteran Affairs website www.va.gov/healthbenefits/online).

2 The list of approved procedures and treatments is *not* identical to Medicare-approved procedures and treatments. They are separate, but clearly, there is substantial overlap. A particular treatment belonging to TFL's approved therapies and not belonging to Medicare's approved treatments is very rare, but there are instances in which this peculiar situation does exist.

3 In this case, a "large employer group plan" is defined as one that covers at least one hundred employees.

4 You can suspend or cancel. If you suspend,

then you can turn on your benefits at a later date. If you cancel, you are canceling permanently. For this reason, FEHB-eligible beneficiaries should choose "suspend."

5 There are unfortunate situations that have occurred and will occur in the future. In Chicago, older retirees are not entitled to premium-free Medicare Part A. That makes the purchase of Medicare Advantage, Medigap, and Part D impossible.

6 Creating High-Quality Results and Outcomes Necessary to Improve Chronic (CHRONIC) Care Act of 2017.

7 This will depend on the specific Medicare Advantage Plan. The Plan carrier will choose, and adjust, which supplementary benefits are available in your geographical area.

Chapter 10

1 If a last-moment legislative change had not been enacted in November 2015, Medicare Part B premiums would have exceeded $152/month for the 30 percent of those not protected by the "hold harmless" provision. The introduction of IRMAA allows the CMS to charge high-income earners more for Medicare Part

B, and the extra amounts being charged are increasing.

2 Distinguishing carriers can be done by only the most experienced, discriminating financial representative. A consumer cannot be expected to know all of the differences because a consumer has only one data point — his or her own.

3 This can also be viewed online: www.cms.gov/medicare/appeals-and-grievances/orgmedffsappeals/index.html.

4 This can be viewed and downloaded online: www.cms.gov/Medicare/Appeals-and-Grievances/MedPrescriptDrugApplGriev/Downloads/Part-D-Late-Enrollment-Penalty-Reconsideration-Request-Form-.pdf.

5 Thirty days if a request for a service, sixty days if the carrier is requesting a payment from you.

6 It is important to use the word "grievance," as it is specific Medicare terminology.

7 This nuance is frequently misunderstood. People receive information from unlicensed personnel and accept it as advice. A licensed person has the fiduciary duty to make suggestions that are in your best interest, irrespective of compensation; "client's interests first" is the standard.

Unlike what you have been likely led to believe, brokers cannot possibly manipulate or alter any price of health insurance, and the idea that "higher premiums mean higher commissions" is patently wrong. Under Medicare Advantage, the compensation rate at a given location will be the same across all of the plans with that same carrier. Unfortunately, it is the case that volunteer-led services frequently attempt to insinuate otherwise.

8 The nuances of this book should be no surprise to a highly qualified professional. (It is not clear that all agents would reach the same conclusions as this book, given the same set of individual circumstances.) This is actually quite important. The market is very competitive, and the only way that you can get the full "bang for your buck" is to know about as many different features as you can and the price of those features.

9 In my practice, I have seen a long list of employers that have wasted a great deal of money when they have Medicare-eligible employees.

Experts' Addendum

1 Genworth Cost of Care Survey 2018, conducted by CareScout®, June 2018

ACKNOWLEDGMENTS

Over the past years, there are a number of people and organizations that have provided support and feedback to me, culminating in this effort.

In no particular order, they are Charles Park, Catherine Johnson, Rachel Shuster, Robert Powell, Norman Harrison, Lewis Seward, Philip Munnerlyn, Sanford J. Mall, Philip Graves, Humana, Inc. (this book is not affiliated with Humana in any way), Hannah Somalski, Sarina Emmendorfer, and Arthur Kuhn. Each has contributed in his or her own specific way that I will not forget.

Like many everyday people, I am dismayed at the crossfire from every angle, on almost every topic in the news cycle. The same can be said about Medicare, where the fragmentation of information is incredible. I simply do not know how a person could practically, confidently, choose by him- or herself. While it is easy to try to find someone else to blame, the fury of complaints has discouraged many from searching out real solutions on this vital topic.

Unfortunately, a great deal of the information regarding Medicare (and other financial matters) comes from people or parties that have never personally met a Medicare beneficiary; they have never put themselves in the shoes of an actual person who is attempting to understand Medicare and make real-world choices. That is the reason that I have included examples with the heading *This Happens.* They are real-life examples. I could not invent them without being there myself, as I have been, in every instance.

Some have suggested that I simply tune out and disassociate from the idea of providing practical answers to practical problems to the general public. I could join a think tank or an insurance carrier, or I could focus solely on wealthy or commercial clients. All have been suggested to me on multiple occasions. I have listened and politely declined these pursuits. There are some specific reasons, specific interactions with people, that have made all the difference.

Jeannie Shene is disabled due to illness

and confined to a wheelchair. She will not walk on her own power, ever. Her attitude could certainly be bitter, angry at the world. That would be understandable; I would probably feel that way. Her illness was purely random. Instead, she set her daily, personal challenges aside and pursued and received my counsel on the best Medicare coverage for her senior parents, one who was seriously ill, without a hint of the hurdles she faces every living day.

Fred Walraven has now passed. He was a well-known farmer in my hometown, a small community in central Michigan. When I explained the options regarding Medicare, he fully understood his age and simply applied his real-world experience as a farmer. He said, "It's always something." He used his common sense and was decisive once he understood the implications of the different plans available. Shortly thereafter, he suffered from brain cancer. Because Fred had secured the highest-quality coverage and had the means to pay for it, the financial consequences of the extensive health care he required were nil. He paid nothing for the months of hospitalization and extensive treatments he received. Fred did not ultimately survive, and while his wife Mary undoubtedly suffered a great deal of stress, thoughts about the financial cost were not on the very long list of concerns she had. Not then, and not now.

The book isn't here solely for you. Someone you know requires intervention, even if unpleasant, even under duress. I guarantee this, 100 percent. Standing by, silent, is convenient; I get it. And while the topic is different, "standing by in silence" is exactly the dynamic that has grown into a cancer afflicting many aspects of our society. We have all looked back and said to ourselves, *I should've said or done something, at that time.* This book is my private attempt at enabling you to do so, now. Share the book or many resources stated in the Introduction. I am certain someone within your tightest circle does not have the information he/she should have to be a savvy Medicare consumer.

INDEX

C

D

E

M

N

O

S

T

U

V

ABOUT THE AUTHOR

Jae W. Oh, MBA, CFP®, CLU®, ChFC®, is the managing principal of GH2 Benefits, LLC, based in Ann Arbor, Michigan. He is a certified financial planner, chartered life underwriter, a chartered financial consultant, and a licensed insurance producer in multiple states.

He is a nationally recognized Medicare expert, frequently quoted in the national press, including on *USA Today,* Dow Jones, CNBC, and Nasdaq.com, as well as on radio talk shows nationwide. He has appeared as a speaker at libraries, for companies, and as part of college-sponsored programs.

Mr. Oh is the founder and current chairman of the Great Humanity Healthcare Foundation, created to provide financial relief to insured persons that are overburdened by medical debt. GH2 Benefits is a full provider of the widest range of financial products and services. Mr. Oh has served in management roles in securities markets on three continents.

He has a master's degree in business administration (MBA) with concentrations in accounting and finance from the University of Chicago and a bachelor of arts (BA) degree in economics and political science from the University of Michigan, Ann Arbor.

You can reach Mr. Oh via the following methods:

Email: jae@maximizeyourmedicare.com
Twitter: www.twitter.com/MaxYourMedicare
Twitter: www.twitter.com/JaeOhCFP
Facebook: www.facebook.com/MaximizeYourMedicare
YouTube: www.youtube.com/maximizeyourmedicare

The employees of Thorndike Press hope you have enjoyed this Large Print book. All our Thorndike, Wheeler, and Kennebec Large Print titles are designed for easy reading, and all our books are made to last. Other Thorndike Press Large Print books are available at your library, through selected bookstores, or directly from us.

For information about titles, please call:

(800) 223-1244

or visit our website at:

gale.com/thorndike

To share your comments, please write:

Publisher
Thorndike Press
10 Water St., Suite 310
Waterville, ME 04901

The employees of Thorndike Press hope you have enjoyed this Large Print book. All our Thorndike, Wheeler, and Kennebec Large Print titles are designed for easy reading, and all our books are made to last. Other Thorndike Press Large Print books are available at your library, through selected bookstores, or directly from us.

For information about titles, please call:
(800) 223-1244

or visit our website at:
gale.com/thorndike

To share your comments, please write:

Publisher
Thorndike Press
10 Water St., Suite 310
Waterville, ME 04901